O P L

OXFORD PSYCHIATRY LIBRARY

Self-Harm

O   P   L
OXFORD PSYCHIATRY LIBRARY

Self-Harm

A Guide to Management

Emmanuel Nii-Boye Quarshie

Senior Lecturer, Department of Psychology
University of Ghana
Legon, Accra
Ghana
and
President, Association for Suicide Prevention Ghana (GASP)
Accra
Ghana

Allan House

Emeritus Professor of Liaison Psychiatry
Leeds Institute of Health Sciences
Worsley Building
University of Leeds
UK

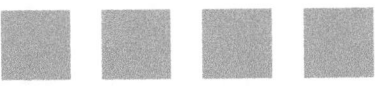

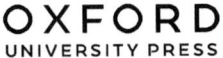

OXFORD
UNIVERSITY PRESS

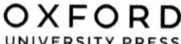

Great Clarendon Street, Oxford, OX2 6DP,
United Kingdom

Oxford University Press is a department of the University of Oxford.
It furthers the University's objective of excellence in research, scholarship,
and education by publishing worldwide. Oxford is a registered trade mark of
Oxford University Press in the UK and in certain other countries

© Oxford University Press 2024

The moral rights of the authors have been asserted

All rights reserved. No part of this publication may be reproduced, stored in
a retrieval system, or transmitted, in any form or by any means, without the
prior permission in writing of Oxford University Press, or as expressly permitted
by law, by licence or under terms agreed with the appropriate reprographics
rights organization. Enquiries concerning reproduction outside the scope of the
above should be sent to the Rights Department, Oxford University Press, at the
address above

You must not circulate this work in any other form
and you must impose this same condition on any acquirer

Published in the United States of America by Oxford University Press
198 Madison Avenue, New York, NY 10016, United States of America

British Library Cataloguing in Publication Data

Data available

Library of Congress Control Number: 2024936387

ISBN 978–0–19–285953–2

DOI: 10.1093/med/9780192859532.001.0001

Printed and bound by
CPI Group (UK) Ltd, Croydon, CR0 4YY

Oxford University Press makes no representation, express or implied, that the
drug dosages in this book are correct. Readers must therefore always check
the product information and clinical procedures with the most up-to-date
published product information and data sheets provided by the manufacturers
and the most recent codes of conduct and safety regulations. The authors and
the publishers do not accept responsibility or legal liability for any errors in the
text or for the misuse or misapplication of material in this work. Except where
otherwise stated, drug dosages and recommendations are for the non-pregnant
adult who is not breast-feeding

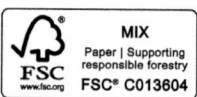

About the authors

Emmanuel Nii-Boye Quarshie is a Senior Lecturer in the Department of Psychology, University of Ghana, Legon, Accra. Nii earned his PhD in Psychological Sciences from the University of Leeds, UK, where he also worked as a Postdoctoral Research Associate at the School of Medicine, Leeds Institute of Health Sciences. Nii remains a Leeds International Research Scholar (LIRS) and has since 2020 been a Visiting Research Fellow in the School of Psychology and the School of Medicine, University of Leeds, UK. He is a Community and Applied Health Psychologist by training, but he also has a strong inclination towards General Psychology. Nii's research focuses on understanding and preventing adolescent self-harm, suicide, and child sexual abuse in low- and middle-income countries (LMICs). He is passionate about developing community-based and in-school interventions to promote adolescent mental health in LMICs, mainly, those within sub-Saharan Africa. He has keen interests in the application of multi-ecological frameworks and interdisciplinary models to understand adolescent self-harm and suicidal behaviours. Nii is the president of the Association for Suicide Prevention Ghana (GASP); he was awarded the prestigious 2021 De Leo Fund Award by the International Association for Suicide Prevention (IASP), for outstanding research on suicidal behaviours carried out in developing countries.

Allan House graduated in medicine in 1974 from St Bartholomew's Hospital, London. After early career positions in hospital medicine and neurology he trained in psychiatry and moved to Leeds in 1989 to work initially as an NHS consultant in liaison psychiatry at Leeds General Infirmary. He was appointed Professor of Liaison Psychiatry in the medical school in Leeds in 1999.

As an academic, Allan's research interests include the interaction between physical illness and mental disorder, medically unexplained syndromes, and self-harm in adults, as well as services for people who present in physical healthcare settings with mental health problems. All his research is planned and delivered in collaboration with people with personal experience of using mental health services.

Allan has published (with colleagues) more than 300 academic papers, and edited or authored five books, all in the area of liaison psychiatry. His recent interests have extended to include the influence of social media on mental health, and the psychiatric perspective on physician-assisted suicide. Details can be found on his university home page https://medicinehealth.leeds.ac.uk/medicine/staff/442/professor-allan-house and his personal blog https://profallanhouse.co.uk/.

Foreword

As an act, self-harm causes both concern and frustration in healthcare. Yet it is still not well understood because it is a complex phenomenon that is not so easy to explain. The academic and clinical dimensions of self-harm are governed by the personal experiences of individuals who struggle to untangle their emotional, behavioural, and social challenges in a very private zone. Because of embarrassment of failing, fear of judgement, and the ordeal to express themselves, the depth of their experiences is obscured.

Also, there is a widespread stigma amongst care providers who respond to self-harm: medically, psychologically, socially and culturally. So there is a need to educate them, equip them with the skills to intervene, and help them develop an effective attitude. An immediate assessment is important to determine an appropriate course of action to help the individual. A particular concern is to identify those who might be at risk of suicide. Because of existing barriers to access services and limited specialist resources, it is crucial that *all* stakeholders in the process are able to respond scientifically.

The challenges of writing a book on self-harm are multiple. An in-depth clinical experience, extensive knowledge of the existing literature and an ability to present it comprehensively to a wide range of audience, living in different parts of the world.

Dr Quarshie has an academic background in psychological sciences with a focus on understanding suicidal behaviour and a strong interest to implement strategies to prevent self-harm in LMICs. His enthusiasm has led him to explore trans-cultural dimensions of self-harm, particularly in adolescents. Prof House is a highly accomplished researcher and an experienced clinician who has learnt the dynamics of self-harm by working directly with people who had lived experiences for over three decades. His contributions towards developing therapeutic interventions to help people with self-harm are highly valuable. Together, they have been able to integrate their knowledge of scientific literature, clinical practice, and diverse cultures to present a much-needed text on self-harm, in a language that can be easily understood by people from different educational backgrounds.

The book can help students of medical, psychological, and social sciences; gatekeepers in the community (teachers, emergency first responders, religious scholars); healthcare providers (at the primary, secondary, and tertiary levels); and most importantly, communities themselves (individuals who are vulnerable to harm themselves and others who wish to support these individuals). It can also guide policymakers and health managers to develop cost-effective services aligned with scientific evidence. Lastly, this book is unique because special attention has been paid to a wide range of social, cultural, and religious aspects of self-harm prevailing across different healthcare contexts.

Dr Asma Humayun, Consultant Psychiatrist
National technical advisor on mental health
Ministry of Planning, Development and Special initiatives, Pakistan

Preface

Self-harm emerged as an area of public health concern and of clinical and academic interest in the second half of the twentieth century—initially mainly in the UK and North America. As its incidence grew dramatically it became clear that it could not be understood simply as an act of attempted suicide that had not, by chance, led to death. Neither could it be fitted into older formulations about, for example, self-mutilation. The modern phenomenon of self-harm can be seen as a symptom of mental disorder, as a response to social or interpersonal stressors— even an adaptive or helpful one at times—or as a sign of individual, intrapersonal, emotional problems arising from earlier life experiences. With the questioning and rethinking of the nature of self-harm, and therefore of the best ways to respond to it, have come changes in terminology. Therapeutic approaches, especially those involving fairly short-term psychological and social interventions, have been developed and tested using rigorous research designs.

Another development in our understanding of self-harm is that in recent years it has become clear that it is not simply restricted to economically developed countries. Rates of self-harm, especially in younger people, approach those in Western Europe and North America and notwithstanding the cultural and social differences in context, many of the features of those at risk are similar in every country where they have been studied.

Despite the amount of research and clinical experience that has evolved in recent years, self-harm remains a significant problem in public health, in mental healthcare, and in terms of the mental and physical wellbeing of individuals. It is still widely misunderstood and stigmatized and as a result many of those affected cannot or will not seek help.

In writing this book, we wanted to produce a brief and accessible summary of what is known about self-harm and its causes. Leading on from this background account we have tried to provide a practical review of what is known about how to respond—at the individual and societal levels—in ways that are based upon research evidence where possible, upon accumulated professional experience and upon the views of those personally affected. We hope you find the result informative and useful.

Acknowledgements

My maiden volume would not have been a success without the love and support of my family, friends, and colleagues at the University of Ghana, particularly Prof Kwaku Oppong Asante. My heartfelt and deepest thanks to Mitch G. Waterman (Professor of Forensic Psychological Science, University of Leeds) and Allan House (Emeritus Professor of Liaison Psychiatry, University of Leeds) from whom I have gained considerable mentorship, knowledge, learning, and inspiration in the area of self-ham and suicide prevention research. I would also like to thank Peter Stevenson—Senior Commissioning Editor, Medicine—Oxford University Press, and Manhar Ghatora—Project Editor, Science and Medical Books—Oxford University Press for their professionalism, patience, and administrative support to get the manuscript to completion.

I am especially grateful to the large number of researchers, authors, and academics whose works have supported and influenced the writing of this book.

ENBQ, Accra, December 2023

I have worked with many people during my clinical and academic career, and I have learned from all of them. Among my longest-standing friends and colleagues with an interest in self-harm I would like to mention particularly Dr David Owens, Prof Nav Kapur, and Prof Mitch Waterman for all the trouble and time they have taken over the years to share ideas, raise questions, and tell me when they think I'm wrong. It is not possible to gain a rounded view of self-harm without discussing ideas and experiences with those with personal experience, and in that regard I would like to thank, for years of informative, critical, and constructive comments, Louise Pembroke and Russell Pembroke.

I would like to join my fellow author Nii in thanking the editorial team at Oxford University Press, and our colleagues Prof Greg Carter and Dr Asma Humayun for taking the time to read and comment on the manuscript. There are of course many others whose ideas and research I have listened to, read, and profited from. They are unfortunately too numerous to name individually, but you will find their works cited throughout this book. My thanks to them all.

AH, Leeds, December 2023

Contents

Part 1
The nature of self-harm
An overview

CHAPTER 1

Definition and terminology

KEY POINTS

- 'Self-harm' and 'attempted suicide' are often used interchangeably and this can cause confusion among researchers, professionals, and lay people.
- The term self-harm is used to describe a person's behaviour rather than their intent.
- Self-harm covers a range of actions, but not everybody agrees how to define or describe it.
- This book defines self-harm as any intentional (non-accidental) act of self-poisoning or self-injury, regardless of the purpose of the act at the time.
- Self-harm can be delineated by referring to three characteristics: method, intent, and lethality.

Definition of self-harm

Not everybody agrees on how to define or describe self-harm and the terms used have changed over time. The World Health Organization, WHO, defines self-harm as '*an act with non-fatal outcome, in which an individual deliberately initiates a non-habitual behaviour that, without intervention from others, will cause self-harm, or deliberately ingests a substance in excess of the prescribed or generally recognised therapeutic dosage, and which is aimed at realising changes which the subject desired via the actual or expected physical consequences*' (Platt et al., 1992).

The WHO definition means that self-harm is intentional, is done by somebody to themselves, and is done by someone who wants to make something change. By saying it is 'non-habitual' it means that it is done as a conscious act, separate from normal day-to-day life.

In this book we adopt a simpler definition for day-to-day use: '*any intentional (non-accidental) act of self-poisoning or self-injury, regardless of the purpose of the act at the time*' (Hawton et al., 2003).

There are two other features that we need to include in our definition. One is that the self-harm falls outside the limits of culturally accepted self-harming activities. Self-harm for our purposes refers to an action that is not seen as normal or usual behaviour, and suggests the individual has problems. We discuss this idea later in the chapter.

Our second exclusion is those behaviours that are undertaken intentionally and have harmful effects but are not undertaken with the primary aim of causing harm—*unintentionally harmful behaviours* such as illicit drug-taking, extreme starvation in anorexia nervosa, or reckless risk-taking. In everyday discussions people often talk about eating disorders as a variety of self-harm, and indeed some of the driving forces are similar—feelings of failure or worthlessness for example. However, it has been usual in psychiatric practice to regard eating disorders as different because they do not have the same immediate and primary aim of harming the individual or the same relation to attempted suicide.

At one time *attempted suicide* was used to describe all acts of self-harm but it leads to a difficulty with clarifying the element of intent, because it does not address the fact that some people who engage in the self-poisoning or self-injury have no clear intention to die (WHO, 2016).

The term *deliberate self-harm* has been widely used but more recently has been seen as problematic. *Deliberate* implies wilfulness and premeditation and is seen as applying a value judgement to the individual involved. For this reason, for example, the UK's Royal College of Psychiatrists says the term *deliberate self-harm* can be seen as offensive or dismissive.

The term *parasuicide* poses a difficulty regarding precise translation. In the languages of some cultures, the prefix 'para' could mean 'mimicking', 'resembling' or 'pretending', which potentially leads to confusion regarding the precise meaning of the behaviour being discussed (WHO, 2016).

In more detail, the definition of self-harm used in this book refers to an act with a non-fatal outcome in which a person does something with the intention of causing harm to themselves. What people do is divided broadly into self-poisoning or self-injury, and occasionally both at the same time (Hawton et al., 2006):

In *self-poisoning*, the individual:

- ingests *(intentionally, non-accidentally)* a medicinal substance in more than the prescribed or generally recognized therapeutic dose.
- ingests a recreational or an illicit drug *with the aim of causing self-harm*[1];
- ingests (by swallowing, inhalation, or sniffing) a substance or object that is usually thought of as non-ingestible, such as acid or pesticide;

In *self-injury*, the individual:

- uses a physical method to 'attack' the body, such as self-cutting, hanging, shooting, strangulation, suffocation, jumping, or throwing self from a height, electrocution, hitting the body or self-battery, burning, drowning;
- undertakes a physical act that results in damage through withdrawal or refusal of something vital—stopping eating (self-starvation), stopping important medication, or other required medical treatment.

---

[1] For illicit/recreational drugs, ingestion of any amount is considered to be in excess of the prescribed or generally recognized therapeutic or effective dose.

To illustrate these ideas, consider a person with Type 1 diabetes who requires insulin treatment to stay well. They might deliberately inject themselves with too much insulin—a form of self-poisoning. They might deliberately refuse to take insulin with the aim of harming themselves—a way of causing self-injury by stopping vital medical treatment. Or they might have discovered that taking too little insulin, or stopping it every so often, is a way of losing weight without having to diet—an action one sometimes sees in people with diabetes and an eating disorder, which is a form of unintentional self-harm.

Because we are interested primarily in self-harm that suggests the individual has social or psychological (mental health) problems, our definition does not include:

- social behaviours that involve ingesting toxic substances that can result in physical or psychological harm, but which are not used for that purpose. This involves actions that may be regarded as socially normal behaviours in many societies such as smoking, recreational drug use, or alcohol consumption;
- Social behaviours that involve injuring the body, such as tattooing or body piercing, for what are often seen as socially normal reasons. These forms of self-injury are usually motivated by a desire to be more attractive or make a social statement rather than by a desire to cause oneself harm;
- intended self-injurious behaviours resulting from religious or tribal ritual or practice—for example, fasting, tribal scarification, manhood rituals, Tatbir. Like the previous example these behaviours may be socially or culturally accepted. They may however be influenced by wider social pressures than the individual choices involved in the examples earlier;
- self-injury or self-poisoning for reasons of political or social protest—such as hunger strikes;
- intended self-injurious behaviours which are not accepted in wider society but are acceptable in the subcultures within which they occur—such as cult groups, or youth subcultures. For example, so-called Goths, Emos or Punks may engage in self-injury as a way of signalling group membership.

Self-harm and suicide

Suicide is many times commoner (up to 50 times commoner) after self-harm than it is in the general population. Unlike repeated self-harm the risk of suicide is not all front-loaded into the first year after self-harm—estimates suggest that over five years after an act of self-harm about 5% of people will die by suicide. Looked at the other way round, more than half of all those who die by suicide have a history of self-harm.

However, the relation between self-harm and suicide is not straightforward. For example, while some people self-harm with a clear intention to die, a person experiencing suicidal thoughts may also self-harm but without the intention to die. In fact, some people self-harm in order to avoid suicide (Edmondson et al., 2016). In other words self-harm and suicide are related and the circumstances that underlie the two behaviours are similar and people who self-harm are at an increased risk of death by suicide, but self-harm is not always intended to lead to death.

All self-harm cannot be regarded as attempted suicide. There is a substantial number of reasons for self-harm other than a desire to die. Broadly speaking they fall into the categories—ways of managing unpleasant emotions, thoughts, or memories; responding to unpleasant emotions, thoughts, or memories without trying to manage or change them; communicating distress, and obtaining positive feelings or self-appraisals from the act (Edmondson et al., 2016). These ideas will be explored further in Chapter 3; in this chapter we will cover only the question of suicidal intent and its presence or absence.

Suicidal intent and self-harm

The definition we are using in this book does not include a statement about suicidal intent and does not therefore divide acts of self-harm according to *suicidal or non-suicidal intent*. This is the approach taken by the WHO and reviewers for the International Cochrane Collaboration (Hawton, Witt, et al., 2015; WHO, 2016). It is at odds with practice in the United States, where the Diagnostic and Statistical Manual of Mental Disorders, Fifth Edition (DSM-5) of the American Psychiatric Association distinguishes between suicidal behaviour and non-suicidal self-injury—often abbreviated to NSSI (APA, 2013).

The US diagnostic practice arises because of a view that it is both important to and possible to distinguish clearly between suicidal and non-suicidal self-harm. In this view, if the intent to die is present to any degree, then the act of self-harm is classified as 'attempted suicide'; the absence of any suicidal intent makes the act 'non-suicidal', unfortunately the DSM terminology identifies explicitly with self-injury only.

The argument for making the distinction is that while both suicidal and non-suicidal self-harm may be risks for later suicide, the two behaviours are different from each other across a number of features apart from intent—course, method, and lethality; demographic characteristics of those involved; and psychosocial variables such as psychiatric diagnosis, impulsivity, or aggression.

One criticism of the DSM-5 classification is that it oversimplifies the distinction, even for a single act. In reality many people who are asked *at the time of an event*—rather than some time afterwards in a clinic or a research study—are unclear or ambiguous about their suicidal intent at the time. Consistently, studies have found that self-injury can be associated with both suicidal and non-suicidal reasons simultaneously. Even within the same episode of self-harm, self-reported intentions can change over minutes or hours. Some people report holding wishes to die and to live simultaneously and indeed one of the stated reasons for apparently non-suicidal self-harm is to help the individual control suicidal impulses

(Edmondson et al., 2016). Muddled or ambivalent descriptions of intent may be particularly likely if somebody has consumed alcohol or drugs during or immediately before an act of self-harm.

Apart from this ambiguity and ambivalence about suicidal intent, it is possible that suicidal intent is deliberately misrepresented by an individual discussing their actions. Some people deny their intent to die—perhaps because of fear of victimization, stigma-related concerns or fear of other repercussions, for example, in countries where suicide is illegal. Occasionally, individuals may feign the intent to die in order to be taken seriously so that they can, for example, obtain access to a mental health service. When an individual feels safe to confide then neither of these misleading responses is common, but the possibility needs to be born in mind especially if there is a possibility of undue pressure from others or a fear of coercive responses from the mental health services.

Although the term non-suicidal self-injury refers to an act, use of the term is often associated with the assumption that the 'non-suicidal' adjective also refers to the person and indeed much clinical and research writing about the topic is based upon that assumption. And yet we know that so-called non-suicidal self-injury is an indication that the individual is at risk for suicide.

For these and related reasons, we do not use terms like 'suicidal ideation' or 'suicidal behaviour' because it is so unclear exactly what they mean (see for example House et al., 2020), and as noted, our definition of self-harm does not include a reference to suicidal intent.

Describing self-harm in further detail

There are two other features of an act of self-harm that should always be included in a full description—the method used, and the act's potential lethality.

Method of self-harm

Conventionally a single act of self-harm is described as self-poisoning, self-injury (for example, cutting, burning, jumping from height) or a mixture of the two. It is important to emphasize that when people self-harm on more than one occasion, using a different method on each occasion is common: that is, somebody who cuts themselves on one occasion is quite likely to take an overdose of tablets on a subsequent occasion.

Both hospital-based and community-based studies have indicated the variety of methods of self-harm used—for example, self-cutting, medication overdose, jumping from a dangerous height such as a bridge or building. In most studies, the commonest methods are self-injury by cutting, and self-poisoning by ingesting prescribed or over-the-counter medication.

Methods of self-harm may differ between countries. Broadly, in high-income countries (including the UK, USA, and Australia) overdose or self-poisoning with medicines and self-cutting are commonly reported. In low- and middle-income countries (including those in Africa, South Asia, and South-East Asia) self-poisoning from pesticides, charcoal burning, drowning, or self-immolation have been reported more commonly. Emerging evidence from sub-Saharan Africa shows that, besides overdose of medicines and poisoning from pesticides, young people ingest household chemicals, including disinfectant and detergents, and cutting is widespread.

Lethality of self-harm

Lethality refers to the biological or medical danger typically related to the method used to self-harm. Violent methods of self-harm such as self-immolation, use of firearms and explosives, drowning, hanging, and jumping from a height, or stepping in front of a moving train or motor vehicle may be considered as having high lethality. Self-poisoning with non-medicinal substances—swallowing bleach or weedkiller for example—can also be considered of high lethality. By contrast scratching, superficial cuts, or overdose of some medications such as benzodiazepines may be considered to be low lethality methods.

Lethality can also be assessed by its physical consequences: the act's physiological consequences and medical procedures required after the self-harm. For example, self-harm that requires inpatient treatment for traumatic injuries or poisoning is typically seen as being of higher lethality than an act that is managed in outpatients or the emergency department only.

It is important to consider the degree of lethality assumed by the individual at the time of the act, especially in relation to self-poisoning. Many people are unaware of the dangers of medications and can either underestimate or overestimate lethality. Because analgesics are readily available for purchase over the counter, an individual may assume a drug like paracetamol is safe even in overdose. On the other hand, because sleeping tablets cause drowsiness then somebody may assume that quite a small overdose of a benzodiazepine will be lethal.

The relation between the lethality of self-harm and suicidal intent is not straightforward. Acts that lead to a need for life-saving treatment have been called *near-fatal self-harm* and are more likely to be associated with suicidal intent, but lethality is only a pointer and cannot be taken as a good test of suicidal intent. While on the face of it all acts of high lethality suggest suicidal intent, the attribution may be incorrect—even acts like these may be undertaken impulsively with little forethought. On the other hand, medically minor episodes like ingesting a small amount of a benzodiazepine sleeping tablet may be associated with a strong wish to die and regret at survival.

Identifying and describing self-harm

Assessment of self-harm helps clarify in detail what has happened leading up to the act and during the act of self-harm. It is also aimed at understanding why somebody has self-harmed (the intent, purpose, or reason for self-harm) and to identify people at risk of repeated self-harm and suicide. A wider assessment will then include, for example, the person's social circumstances and mental state. We will discuss the full assessment of self-harm later, in Chapter 7. Here we consider some common approaches to defining the act and clarifying suicidal intent.

Describing the act

The first step in assessment is to clarify what happened and when. At its simplest this can involve only one or two questions to establish that self-harm (as defined here) has taken place. This needs to be done in an individually and culturally sensitive way: if initial answers remain unclear, more detail can be obtained by asking the person to describe in their own words what happened and when.

The advantage of this sort of informal interviewing style is that it can put the person at ease, helping them feel they are in control of the situation and therefore talk more freely. The disadvantage is that important information may be missed because the questioning is not standardized. For this reason, more structured and standardized approaches can be used, especially in research. An example is the Suicide Attempt Self-Injury Interview (SASII) which is widely employed in research assessments. It has the advantage of being comprehensive but is unlikely to be realistic in settings where a distressed person is discussing their self-harm perhaps for the first time. We mention it here because, for those unfamiliar with self-harm, it can provide useful pointers for topics that might come up in an informal interview.

Assessing suicide intent

Having assessed the nature and timing of an act of self-harm including the method used and its potential lethality, the other important question raised by this introductory chapter is the suicidal intent associated with the act. Again, at its simplest it is possible to ask a single question about desire or intention to die at the time of, and as a result of, the self-harm. However, there is a real risk in asking a question that requires a Yes or No answer when the individual may have mixed views about suicide that change over time or may have been unclear at the time about their intentions. It is better to explore in more detail, accepting that intent is unlikely to be an all-or-nothing attitude to living or dying. In relation to a particular act of self-harm, a useful template is provided by Beck's Suicide Intent Scale (Beck et al., 1974) which distinguishes between self-reported intent and circumstances of an act of self-harm that give pointers towards intent (see Table 1.1).

The motivation or intention of self-harm cannot be assumed based on the method of self-harm used so it should not be assumed, for example, that because somebody has cut themselves then the motive for the act is non-suicidal.

Even more importantly, assessment should not confuse the suicidal intent of a particular episode of self-harm with the suicidal risk of the individual being assessed. So-called non-suicidal self-harm is associated with a substantially elevated risk of hospital re-admission and a 2- to 5-fold increased risk of subsequent suicide death compared to the general population (Birtwistle et al., 2017). One explanation for this is that self-harm is used by some people as a way of keeping suicidal thoughts at bay, for example, by inflicting pain or punishment.

Table 1.1 Features to consider in assessing suicidal intent (from Beck SIS)	
Circumstances of the act	Self-report
• Isolation • Timing (likelihood of intervention) • Precautions against discovery/intervention • Acting to get help during/after attempt • Final acts in anticipation of death (will, gifts, insurance) • Active preparation for attempt • Suicide note • Overt communication of intent before the attempt	• Reported purpose of attempt • Expectations of fatality • Conception of method's lethality • Seriousness of attempt • Attitude toward living/dying • Conception of medical rescuability with treatment • Degree of premeditation

Even though the relationship between the lethality of self-harm method and suicide intention is unclear and inconsistent, knowing the self-harm method is useful in the assessment of people presenting with self-harm. Knowing what methods people use to self-harm is also helpful in developing strategies to prevent self-harm—whether in the clinic, workplace, school, prison, household, or within the general community context.

Implications for practice

The first part of the assessment of self-harm involves finding out exactly what happened—the circumstances of the act, the method used, and its potential lethality. There are many reasons for self-harm, to be discussed later in this book: an immediate question for assessment is to determine the degree of suicidal intent in the act.

Interviews involve an in-person, virtual, or telephone discussion. In-person (face-to-face) interviews are best but not always achievable; for example, if there are severe restrictions on travel to meet up. This approach yields first-hand responses about the nature, timing, motivation, and circumstances of self-harm, and is the best general approach. Care needs to be taken to obtain a full picture and it is important to be aware that some people may provide socially desirable or evasive answers because of fear of the consequences if they are too open about how they feel.

Self-report approaches involve giving out self-report questionnaires or behavioural checklists. They have the advantage that a structured approach means it is clear what areas have been covered, and their relatively anonymous or bureaucratic nature may make it easier for respondents to distance themselves emotionally from the issues and therefore answer more directly about what has happened. On the other hand, some people find filling out forms off-putting and are more likely to hold back than they are in relaxed interview. They are less useful in settings where levels of general or health literacy are low.

The exact approach to assessment will depend upon circumstances—the time available, the willingness of the respondents to explain what happened, the relationship between the person doing the assessment, and the person being assessed. A mixture of interview and standardized questionnaire might be considered ideal to obtain a full picture, but in reality an interview covering the main points in this chapter is likely to be the most realistic in most settings.

Assessment after self-harm involves more than deciding what exactly has happened and with what suicidal intent. We will return to discuss these wider aspects of assessment in Chapter 7.

In summary:

- Self-harm may involve self-poisoning, self-injury, or a mixture of both.
- An initial assessment may involve interview or standardized questionnaires.
- An important start to assessment is to determine the circumstances of self-harm and what method was used, including its potential lethality.
- Suicidal intent should not be treated as simply present or absent: it may fluctuate, the respondent may be unclear or simultaneously have wished to die and to survive.
- The circumstances of an act, as well as reported reasons for self-harm, can help with assessment of suicidal intent.

REFERENCES

APA (2013). *Diagnostic and statistical manual of mental disorders* (5th ed.). Washington, DC: American Psychiatric Publishing.

Beck, A. T., Schuyler, D., & Herman, I. (1974). Development of suicidal intent scales. In A. T. Beck, H. L. P. Resnik, & D. J. Lettieri (Eds.), *The prediction of suicide* (pp. 45–58). Bowie, MD: Charles Press.

Birtwistle, J., Kelley, R., House, A., & Owens, D. (2017). Combination of self-harm methods and fatal and non-fatal repetition: a cohort study. *Journal of Affective Disorders, 218*, 188–194. https://doi.org/10.1016/j.jad.2017.04.027

Edmondson, A. J., Brennan, C. A., & House, A. O. (2016). Non-suicidal reasons for self-harm: a systematic review of self-reported accounts. *Journal of Affective Disorders, 191*, 109–117. https://doi.org/10.1016/j.jad.2015.11.043

Hawton, K., Harriss, L., Hall, S., Simkin, S., Bale, E., & Bond, A. (2003). Deliberate self-harm in Oxford, 1990–2000: a time of change in patient characteristics. *Psychological Medicine, 33*(6), 987–995. https://doi.org/10.1017/S0033291703007943

Hawton, K., Rodham, K., & Evans, E. (2006). *By their own young hand: deliberate self-harm and suicidal ideas in adolescents*. London: Jessica Kingsley Publishers.

Hawton, K., Witt, K. G., Salisbury, T. L. T., Arensman, E., Gunnell, D., Townsend, E., van Heeringen, K., & Hazell, P. (2015). Interventions for self-harm in children and adolescents. *Cochrane Database of Systematic Reviews*, (12), 1–105. https://doi.org/10.1002/14651858.CD012013

House, A., Kapur, N., & Knipe, D. (2020). Thinking about suicidal thinking. *The Lancet Psychiatry*, 7(11), 997–1000. https://doi.org/10.1016/S2215-0366(20)30263-7

Platt, S., Bille-Brahe, U., Kerkhof, A., Schmidtke, A., Bjerke, T., Crepet, P., Leo, D. D., Haring, C., Lonnqvist, J., & Michel, K. (1992). Parasiticide in Europe: the WHO/EURO multicentre study on parasuicide. I. Introduction and preliminary analysis for 1989. *Acta Psychiatrica Scandinavica*, 85(2), 97–104. https://doi.org/10.1111/j.1600-0447.1992.tb01451.x

WHO (2016). *Practice manual for establishing and maintaining surveillance systems for suicide attempts and self-harm*. WHO.

CHAPTER 2

Self-harm: The nature of the problem

KEY POINTS

- Much of what is known about self-harm comes from research conducted in high-income countries.
- Self-harm is common in the community, with most persons who self-harm not presenting to clinical care.
- Self-harm occurs most commonly in adolescence, but self-harm is not uncommon throughout the lifespan.
- Females are more likely than males to report self-harm.

How common is self-harm?

The challenge of measurement

There is no simple, straightforward way to answer the question: 'how common is self-harm?' The answer depends on several factors, including of course how self-harm is defined: whether the interest is in self-harm without regard to the intent of the act or only in attempted suicide, or only in self-harm with purposes other than suicide. Another relevant part of the definition is the *method of self-harm*—whether self-injury (such as cutting), self-poisoning, or both. These definitional issues are covered in Chapter 1.

Other important influences on the answer are:

The population of interest—for example, whether people were identified because they contacted clinical services—outpatients, inpatients or patients presenting to emergency department, or because they were part of minority groups, indigenous people, or the general population;

The age of informants—whether the interest is in self-harm among children, adolescents, or adults;

The time frame—whether the focus is a current act of self-harm, the past 6 or 12 months, or across the course of a lifetime;

The geographical location—whether interest is in particular national, regional, continental figures, or in the global situation. Much of what is known about self-harm during the past half a century, including how common it is, comes from research conducted in high-income countries, particularly those in Europe, Oceania, and North America. Research in low- and middle-income countries has only started recently, as the problem is now coming to the attention of parents, families, health professionals, teachers, social workers, and religious leaders who are in frequent contact with those most likely to self-harm, whether young or old.

Sources of information

Information about how common self-harm is can be obtained through two primary sources: medical records that catalogue self-harm presenting to *clinical services*, and self-reports of self-harm in *research surveys* of representative samples of the population.

Research from many countries in both high-income and low- and middle-income contexts indicates that self-harm is common in the community especially among young people, most of whom do not present to clinical care. For example, only one in eight adolescents who self-harm presents to a clinic or hospital. Reasons vary but it is likely that an important reason is shame and fear of being judged critically by other people, including hospital staff. Another common reason for non-presentation is concern that seeking clinical help will lead to others finding out about self-harm—family, friends, school, or employers for example.

When people do present to healthcare after acts of self-harm, it is likely to be because the act requires immediate medical treatment—perhaps it involved the use of potentially lethal methods such as a drug overdose, or a self-inflicted wound that will not stop bleeding or has become infected. Sometimes medical treatment is sought but the reasons for it are disguised—for example, being misrepresented as an accident. The implication is that information collected about self-harm from clinics and hospitals may not be a true reflection of the complete picture of the behaviour.

Similarly, surveys conducted in the general community or in specific locations like schools are likely to underestimate the frequency of self-harm—owing to the shame and stigma associated with the behaviour, participants may provide socially desirable and guarded answers to questions related to self-harm. This is especially likely where the research is taking place in a country where self-harm or attempted suicide is difficult to discuss because of religious prohibitions, or suicide is a crime and police involvement may follow.

Frequency of self-harm in the general population

A note on terminology

The frequency of a condition is usually expressed in one of two ways, as *prevalence* or *incidence*. Prevalence is probably the more familiar idea. It simply tells us what proportion of a group of people has a particular condition; for example, what percentage of the adult population has diabetes, or smokes cigarettes. So, prevalence is expressed simply as a fraction; as a percentage for common problems, as a number per thousand, ten thousand, or even million for rare problems. Incidence tells us about how frequent new cases are; for example, how many people in a particular population have a heart attack each year. So, when incidence is expressed the figure includes a time period as well: for example, the suicide rate in England and Wales is approximately 10 per 100,000 population per year. This is the annual incidence. For a very common condition, for example new cases of COVID-19 infection during the recent pandemic, incidence might be expressed as weekly or even daily new cases. Self-harm is one of those conditions that may occur repeatedly. In that case, incidence is typically calculated by taking only the individual's first act within the time period, so it is the incidence of new people presenting with an episode rather than new episodes.

When prevalence is recorded at a particular time, as in the example just given, it is known as the *point prevalence*. This is fine for a chronic condition like diabetes but it doesn't make sense for an episodic behaviour like self-harm. Instead, it is usual to report what is called a *period prevalence*—for example, telling us what proportion of people in a given population have self-harmed in the last 6 months, or ever in their life (lifetime prevalence).

Frequency of self-harm

Only a few major international studies (including Weissman et al., 1999; Bertolote et al., 2005) have explored the frequency of self-harm in the general population (all ages or adults only). Methods, including the questions asked to elicit a history of self-harm, varied but the results are relatively consistent. They show that, as a reasonable approximation, about 4–5% of the population have at some time in their life undertaken an act described as attempted suicide. The prevalence of all acts of self-harm, included regardless of stated intent, is likely to be significantly higher and perhaps double that figure.

There are striking international differences in the figures, with findings in countries where self-harm is commonest being ten times what they are in the countries where self-harm is least common. As a generalization it appears that self-harm is commonest in economically developed countries of Europe, North America, and Oceania. However, caution is needed in assuming this pattern is fixed; a review of recent studies from sub-Saharan Africa suggested that the prevalence of self-harm in young people is similar to that in higher-income countries, and it must be assumed that the phenomenon of self-harm exists in every part of the world and is likely to be under-recognized in most countries.

Repeated self-harm is common and something like a quarter to a third of people (25–30%) who have self-harmed at all have done it more than once. Young people who self-harm are more likely to have a history of repeated episodes. In a large sample of 22,910 individuals (aged 10 years or older) who had self-harmed and presented to hospital emergency departments in Northern Ireland from April 2012 to March 2017, 41% re-presented to the emergency departments following further self-harm in the next 12 months (Griffin et al., 2019). Findings from an international survey of community and school samples of adolescents (mainly 15–16-year-olds) across Europe and Australia indicate that just over half of the adolescents who self-harmed during the previous year also reported multiple episodes (Madge et al., 2008). Similar community-based evidence has been reported recently from Ghana (in sub-Saharan Africa), where 50% of in-school and street-connected adolescents who met the criteria for self-harm during the past 12 months reported more than one episode over their lifetime (Quarshie et al., 2021).

It is useful to draw the distinction between self-harm that happens in response to acute distress and self-harm that occurs repeatedly in relation to enduring unresolved adverse life circumstances or emotional distress. The risk factors for self-harm and its repetition are discussed in Chapter 3 of this book; here it is simply worth noting that long-standing, unresolved adverse psychological and social factors are the most consistent risks for repeated self-harm, while for some people self-harm is a response to a specific life event or problem and may not repeat once the immediate problem is resolved.

Self-harm across the lifespan

Children

There are few studies of self-harm in children younger than 12 years. School and community-based studies have reported only scant evidence on self-harm among younger children, and the presentations of self-harm to health facilities hardly involve individuals in this younger age group.

At least two hospital-based studies have been conducted. Marraccini and colleagues analysed medical records of 502 children and adolescents aged 6–18 years admitted to a psychiatric inpatient hospital in the United States between 2015 and 2018 for suicide-related risk: 121 were children aged 6–12 years and 32 (26%) of these children reported an episode of self-harm (Marraccini et al., 2021). The Multicentre Study of Self-harm in England monitors contacts for self-harm in five hospitals. In the years 2000–2016, 387 children aged 5–12 years presented to the study hospitals, 39% of whom were 5–11 years (Geulayov et al., 2022). Clearly the numbers are small but in children so young, they are concerning.

Adolescents

Self-harm in adolescents has attracted much more attention. Recent systematic reviews of longitudinal studies suggest that self-harm is common during adolescence, around mid-ages 15–16 years and declines towards late-ages 18–19 years to early adulthood.

Research findings from Western countries suggest that the highest rates of hospital-treated self-harm are reported among young people. Some 40–60% of adolescent psychiatric inpatients have self-harmed during the previous 12 months, while 20% of adolescents approached in a community or school context report self-harm in the past year. Taken together, the evidence suggests that, before attaining age 19, 20% or more of young people in Western contexts have self-harmed at least once.

Interestingly, emerging research findings from low- and middle-income countries show that the prevalence estimates of self-harm among adolescents within the region are comparable. For example, estimates indicate that between 11% and 25% of young people from sub-Saharan Africa report a history of self-harm during the previous 12 months (Quarshie et al., 2020). As noted earlier, about half of adolescents who have self-harmed at all have done so more than once, a finding that is in line with a recent review of all studies of repeated self-harm (two or more episodes) which found a lifetime prevalence of just under 5%, with huge variation between countries, from 1 to 14% (Smith et al., 2022).

It appears that across the world there are significant societal changes that are likely to affect the mental health of young people. These changes are linked to globalization so that similar economic, social, and environmental stresses come to affect young people in many countries: as a result self-harm as a culturally understood phenomenon becomes more familiar. There remain, however, substantial differences between countries in rates of self-harm in adolescents.

Adults

International estimates are that lifetime prevalence of self-harm is about 1 out of 10 young adults, and 1 out of 20 people in middle age. There are few data on the lifetime prevalence of self-harm in older adults, but the 12-month prevalence is much lower than in adolescents and younger adult life; 1 in 1000 or fewer older adults report self-harm in the preceding year (Troya et al., 2019).

Reasons for age-related differences

Adolescence is a period of human development in which rapid brain maturation and puberty lead to new sets of capacities and behaviours that set-in motion or enable transitions in family relationships, friendship, and educational domains, and in health behaviours. The relatively higher occurrence of self-harm during adolescence and the striking association with puberty has been attributed partly to neuro-developmental vulnerability during adolescence, with elevated chances of risk-taking behaviours and emotional disorders.

Adolescents are relatively more vulnerable to adverse social and interpersonal events such as rejection by peers, and many adolescents feel pressured to meet the expectations of others, including families, parents, peers, and teachers. Problem-solving capacities are less developed during this period; adolescents are much more likely to experience depression, anxiety, and esteem issues. Many do not seek help from family or formal support sources but may confide in friends, while some respond to emotional distress by drinking alcohol, smoking, or (mis)using recreational drugs. Given the complex nature of this period of development, many adolescents may feel overwhelmed in the face of problems in life.

It is not clear why self-harm is less common during adulthood. Perhaps life settles down and presents fewer challenges as people get older. Also, it is possible that over time people learn through life experiences and find more effective and efficient ways of responding to emotional distress and unpleasant circumstances.

Older adults who self-harm have some distinguishing characteristics—for example, stressful physical illness, heightened loneliness associated either with bereavement or with difficulties leaving the house, loss of control, previous and current psychiatric problems, and perceived burdensomeness.

Self-harm and gender

There is a striking relationship between gender and self-harm. In the UK study noted earlier, among children aged 5–12 years who presented to the study hospitals boys outnumbered girls two to one at ages 5–10 years: the numbers of boys and girls who self-harmed were similar at age 11, while at age 12 there were nearly four girls to every boy (Geulayov et al., 2022).

Studies from many parts of the world find that self-harm is more frequent among females than males. Community and school-based surveys from Europe, Australia, and North America have shown that girls are about 2 to 3 times more likely than boys to report self-harm. A recent study of emergency department attendance in the UK suggests that for self-harm among adolescents aged 12–14 years, girls outnumber boys 6 to 1 (Diggins et al., 2017).

It has also been observed that by early adulthood the rate among females drops to a comparable level with that of males—even though they still remain slightly higher in females (Diggins et al., 2017). Presentations to hospital emergency departments in Ireland by young people aged 10–24 years during the period 2007–2016 were 368 per 100,000 females and 271 per 100,000 males (Griffin et al., 2018).

Very little is known from prospective studies about the natural history of self-harm in relation to gender among the general adult population. Even though research findings on self-harm in low- and middle-income countries are still sparse, recent syntheses of reported research evidence are also showing that in young people self-harm is more frequently reported among females than males (Quarshie et al., 2020).

The consistent finding that rates of self-harm are higher in females than males is difficult to explain. It has been suggested that men and boys are more reluctant than women and girls to report self-harm, perhaps misconstruing such an admission as a threat to their sense of masculinity. Additionally, some injuries—for example, from punching walls or head banging—that lead boys to hospital are more easily reported as accidents than the self-harm (overdose, cutting, or burning) that takes girls into accident and emergency departments, so clinical data may also under-represent the extent of the problem of self-harm in boys.

The gender difference in rates of self-harm in adolescents has been partly attributed to the different physical make-up of boys and girls during puberty. Girls generally reach puberty earlier than boys. Findings from brain biochemistry, twin, family, and adoption studies have suggested that puberty may bring with it the activation of genetically predetermined vulnerabilities to self-harm and suicidal behaviours. Pubertal maturation begins in the brain, with some neural changes leading to hormonal increases in early puberty. Brain maturation progresses well into late adolescence and emerging adulthood, particularly, in regions of the brain connected to regulation of emotions and behaviour. These progressive brain changes correlate with the development of response inhibition, mature judgement, attentional regulation, and self-control, and continue beyond the next decade after the onset of puberty. Thus, early maturers may experience a developmental gap between puberty and brain development; immature emotional control, poor judgement, and patterns of social adversity may influence the rate and form of self-harm in early adolescent girls than boys. In a recent publication drawing on the birth cohort study the Avon Longitudinal Study of Parents and Children (ALSPAC) in the UK, researchers found that early menarche (at age 11.5 years or younger) was associated with an increased risk of self-harm, whereas later menarche (at age 13.8 years or older) was associated with a reduced risk of self-harm (Roberts et al., 2020).

There is good reason to believe that puberty and related neurodevelopmental vulnerability may not be adequate in accounting for the large and persistent gender difference in the rates of self-harm. For example, genetic research suggests that, at best, the contributions of heredity to mood disorders does not exceed 40% (Patel, 2013), supporting the idea that environmental and social factors may be playing a stronger role in explaining the gender and individual differences in the rates of mood disorders (and by extension, self-harm) in young people.

Environmental influences, such as peer interactions and influences, appear to be particularly effective in creating 'hot cognitions' (thinking under conditions of high arousal or strong emotion) and such states may also be related to impulsive tendencies and an increased risk of self-directed harmful behaviours. It is possible that the association between puberty and self-harm is activated and compounded by the (earlier) presence of social adversities. For example, there is evidence to suggest that childhood sexual abuse and other childhood adversities including family conflict may be associated with early menarche.

Most of the factors associated with self-harm as risks and protective variables have been identified within the social environment and psychological domains, particularly negative emotional experiences and processes. More recently, leading researchers have linked the high frequency of self-harm in girls to contemporary increases in psychological distress, including emotional pressures emanating from social media experienced mostly by girls.

In low- and middle-income countries (particularly those in Africa, the Caribbean, and South Asia), the higher rates of self-harm in adolescent girls than boys have been attributed to the entrenched and exploitative normative gender role discrimination against girls and women. Relative to boys, girls tend to be burdened with more domestic chores, overwhelming caretaking responsibilities, and are victims of sexual abuse and exploitation, early marriage, exclusion from education and recreational activities such as sports, unemployment, social isolation, and exclusion from decision-making. Thus, these rigid gender norms and discrimination, plus the natural increased risk of emotional problems during puberty, increase the chances that more girls than boys will self-harm.

Mental disorder and self-harm

Although self-harm is best understood as a response to societal, interpersonal, and personal circumstances, it can occasionally be seen as a symptom of mental disorder. Although not common except in hospital settings, self-harm associated with mental disorders is especially important because it is more likely to be associated with suicidal intent.

Pretty much any mental disorder may be associated with self-harm, but for obvious reasons the most common are those disorders associated with depressive symptoms and related ideas such as worthlessness, hopelessness, guilt, or a sense of failure. This includes bipolar disorder, eating disorders, anxiety disorders, and obsessional disorders. Psychotic disorders are relatively rarely encountered, although very occasionally self-harm may be a response to delusional thinking, such as a belief in a need for punishment.

Mental disorders should be considered, and especially carefully sought, when self-harm occurs for the first time in middle or later adult life.

Other demographic, social, and cultural features of those who self-harm

In summary, there are certainly differences in the frequency of self-harm so that it appears commonest in young people and especially females, and in higher-income countries. Nonetheless, the overall picture that emerges is that self-harm can occur at any age, in both genders, and in every country or region in which it has been studied. Against this background, there are groups of people in every society who appear to be at greater risk of self-harm. These include:

- Minority groups whose members are discriminated against in society, such as racial or ethnic minorities, gender, and sexual minorities. Discrimination can have consequences that are emotional (fear, distress) social (rejection by peers or family) or practical and social (exclusion from employment or housing). At the same time, it can restrict access to informal support and to helping agencies, especially where official policy is discriminatory.
- People from economically disadvantaged backgrounds or of low socio-economic status, for whom social problems are compounded by lack of resources to respond effectively.

- People with physical and mental disabilities. Unfortunately, in many countries people with disabilities are discriminated against and at the same time they have fewer employment opportunities and therefore more financial problems. Disabilities such as immobility and learning disability may severely limit capacity to respond effectively to these increased challenges.

- People living with life-limiting and other severe and chronic health conditions such as cancer, stroke, HIV/AIDS, and end-stage renal disease. Such illnesses, especially if they are associated with symptoms such as pain, breathlessness, and sleep disturbance, can readily lead to depression and a sense of hopelessness.

- Prisoners (including young offenders). Prisons can be threatening places, where intimidation is common and drug use is a widespread response to lack of physical and mental activity. Overcrowding, in itself stressful, may be accompanied by a lack of social and emotional support.

- Asylum-seekers, refugees, and persons living in fragile social contexts, including war-torn areas. In addition to the ever-present sense of threat, people in these situations have often been disrupted from their usual social and cultural ties and therefore lack support of all sorts—emotional and practical.

- Workers in certain categories of occupation are also likely to self-harm (including farmers, military, police, and other first responders). The reasons are not clear—perhaps availability of means, occupational exposure to non-natural death, or a culture that does not encourage sharing of emotional problems.

Implications for practice

Self-harm is found across all societies and its existence should be discussed with concern but without undue alarm or negative judgements.

Those working in education should be especially aware of how common self-harm is among young people, especially girls and young women, and be willing to discuss it if it comes to attention.

Those who encounter members of other vulnerable groups, through paid employment or charitable work, should be aware of how common self-harm is, and be willing to discuss it openly if it comes to attention.

Public health measures aimed at reducing self-harm, both for its own sake and as an important part of a suicide prevention strategy, will need to take account of the general population picture and also of high-risk groups for whom specific targeted interventions may be helpful.

In summary

- Self-harm is reported in all societies in which it has been studied, although it appears commonest in high-income countries.
- Approximately 5% of people have self-harmed at some time, and for the highest risk groups the rate may be as high as 25% or more,
- Self-harm is commoner among females than males, and in adolescence and young adulthood.
- Self-harm is common in vulnerable groups who experience discrimination, social, and personal adversity, live with severe illness or disabilities, and those who are cut off from social support.
- Social adversities and life problems (rather than the different biological make-up) of females and males provide a good basis to explain the gender differences in the rates.

REFERENCES

Bertolote, J. M., Fleischmann, A., De Leo, D., Bolhari, J., Botega, N., De Silva, D., Thanh, H. T. T., Phillips, M., Schlebusch, L., & Värnik, A. (2005). Suicide attempts, plans, and ideation in culturally diverse sites: the WHO SUPRE-MISS community survey. *Psychological Medicine*, *35*(10), 1457–1465. https://doi.org/10.1017/S003329170 5005404

Diggins, E., Kelley, R., Cottrell, D., House, A., & Owens, D. (2017). Age-related differences in self-harm presentations and subsequent management of adolescents and young adults at the emergency department. *Journal of Affective Disorders*, *208*, 399–405. https://doi.org/10.1016/j.jad.2016.10.014

Geulayov, G., Casey, D., Bale, L., Brand, F., Townsend, E., Ness, J., Rehman, M., Waters, K., Clements, C., & Farooq, B. (2022). Self-harm in children 12 years and younger: characteristics and outcomes based on the Multicentre Study of Self-harm in England. *Social Psychiatry and Psychiatric Epidemiology*, *57*, 139–148. https://doi.org/10.1007/s00 127-021-02133-6

Griffin, E., Bonner, B., O'Hagan, D., Kavalidou, K., & Corcoran, P. (2019). Hospital-presenting self-harm and ideation: comparison of incidence, profile and risk of repetition. *General Hospital Psychiatry*, *61*, 76–81. https://doi.org/10.1016/j.genhospps ych.2019.10.009

Griffin, E., McMahon, E., McNicholas, F., Corcoran, P., Perry, I. J., & Arensman, E. (2018). Increasing rates of self-harm among children, adolescents and young adults: a 10-year national registry study 2007–2016. *Social Psychiatry and Psychiatric Epidemiology*, *53*(7), 663–671. https://doi.org/10.1007/s00127-018-1522-1

Madge, N., Hewitt, A., Hawton, K., Wilde, E. J. D., Corcoran, P., Fekete, S., Heeringen, K. V., Leo, D. D., & Ystgaard, M. (2008). Deliberate self-harm within an international community sample of young people: comparative findings from the Child & Adolescent Self-harm in Europe (CASE) Study. *Journal of Child Psychology and Psychiatry*, *49*(6), 667–677. https://doi.org/10.1111/j.1469-7610.2008.01879.x

Marraccini, M. E., Drapeau, C. W., Stein, R., Pittleman, C., Toole, E. N., Kolstad, M., Tow, A. C., & Suldo, S. M. (2021). Characterizing children hospitalized for suicide-related thoughts and behaviors. *Child and Adolescent Mental Health*, 26(4), 331–338. https://doi.org/10.1111/camh.12454

Patel, V. (2013). Reducing the burden of depression in youth: what are the implications of neuroscience and genetics on policies and programs? *Journal of Adolescent Health*, 52(2), S36–S38. https://doi.org/10.1016/j.jadohealth.2012.04.016

Quarshie, E. N.-B., Shuweihdi, F., Waterman, M., & House, A. (2021). Self-harm among in-school and street-connected adolescents in Ghana: a cross-sectional survey in the Greater Accra region. *BMJ Open*, 0:e041609. https://doi.org/10.1136/bmjopen-2020-041609

Quarshie, E. N.-B., Waterman, M. G., & House, A. O. (2020). Self-harm with suicidal and non-suicidal intent in young people in sub-Saharan Africa: a systematic review. *BMC Psychiatry*, 20(234), 1–26. https://doi.org/10.1186/s12888-020-02587-z

Roberts, E., Fraser, A., Gunnell, D., Joinson, C., & Mars, B. (2020). Timing of menarche and self-harm in adolescence and adulthood: a population-based cohort study. *Psychological Medicine*, 50(12), 2010–2018. https://doi.org/10.1017/S0033329171 9002095

Smith, L., Shin, J., Carmichael, C., et al. (2022). Prevalence and correlates of multiple suicide attempts among adolescents aged 12-15 years from 61 countries in Africa, Asia, the Americas. *Journal of Psychiatric Research*, 144, 45–53. https://doi.org/10.1016/j.psychres.2021.09.047

Troya, M. I., Babatunde, O., Polidano, K., Bartlam, B., McCloskey, E., Dikomitis, L., & Chew-Graham, C. A. (2019). Self-harm in older adults: systematic review. *The British Journal of Psychiatry*, 214(4), 186–200. https://doi.org/10.1192/bjp.2019.11

Weissman, M. M., Bland, R. C., Canino, G. J., Greenwald, S., Hwu, H.-G., Joyce, P. R., Karam, E. G., Lee, C.-K., Lellouch, J., & Lepine, J.-P. (1999). Prevalence of suicide ideation and suicide attempts in nine countries. *Psychological Medicine*, 29(1), 9–17. https://doi.org/10.1017/S0033291798007867

Understanding the reasons for self-harm

KEY POINTS

- People often report multiple reasons for their self-harm.
- The intention of self-harm cannot be assumed based on the method of self-harm used.
- Non-suicidal reasons for self-harm are mostly related to responding to distress.
- Self-harm is mostly not confided in others.
- Repeated self-harm is not 'manipulative' or 'attention-seeking'.

What are the common psychological and social risks for self-harm?

Self-harm is complex and cannot be attributed to a single risk or cause. This means that there is no straightforward single answer to a question about why someone has self-harmed—an explanation needs to be more like a story leading to the outcome of self-harm than a description of a single factor explaining the act. Risks are different for young people and adults (see Table 3.1). When asked about reasons for an episode of self-harm, people usually answer in one of three ways. First, they may mention problems or worries arising from the community in which they live. Second, they may describe personal, individual problems—for example, how they feel emotionally or difficulties they are having with thinking about how to tackle problems. Third, and most commonly, they may outline problems in their immediate social network—with family, friends, or romantic relationships.

Viewing self-harm in this way has been called using a *socioecological model*, where risk and protective factors are considered at the wider community, individual, and relational levels. The common risk factors in self-harm are shown in Table 3.1.

What reasons do people report for their self-harm?

A question remains however: given that somebody describes these problems, why is it that self-harm is their response? As mentioned earlier in Chapter 1, self-harm may serve several purposes or functions and many people who engage in

Table 3.1 Common risks and factors associated with self-harm

At risk groups

- Minority, migratory, and marginalized groups (including sexual and gender minority groups, indigenous populations, ethnic minority groups, refugees, internally displaced persons, and asylum seekers)
- Low socioeconomic status (including unemployment, family poverty, financial problems, homelessness, and street-living)
- Prisoners (including juvenile justice involved young people)
- Foster, kinship, or institutional care
- Adverse childhood experiences

Problematic current circumstances

- Social isolation (including lack of close friends)
- Hunger (food deprivation)**
- Poor schoolwork (poor academic performance)**
- Access to means of self-harm
- Exposure to self-harm by friends and/or family members*

Individual characteristics

Mental health problems

- Personal history of self-harm
- Suicidal thinking
- Mental disorders (commonly depression, eating disorders, anxiety. Less commonly attention deficit hyperactivity disorder*, autism spectrum disorder, dissociative disorder, psychosis)
- Drugs and alcohol (mis)use

Psychological characteristics

- physical health problems and disability (including chronic physical pain)***
- Loss of sense of personal control***
- Increased sense of burdensomeness***
- Impulsivity*
- Low self-esteem*
- Hopelessness and despair
- Poor social problem-solving skills (including poor communication skills)
- Regret about missed opportunities***

Recent stressful experiences

- Bereavement [including death of parent(s)*, and bereavement by suicide]
- Romantic relationship breakup*
- Parental divorce or separation*
- Parental neglect*
- Conflict with parents*
- Child marriage (girls)**
- Household and community violence (including emotional, sexual, or physical abuse)
- Bullying victimization* including on social media (cyberbullying victimization)*
- Unwanted pregnancy (teenage pregnancy)**

* Young people; ** young people in low and middle-income countries; *** among older adults.

self-harm report multiple reasons for the act. There is a substantial number of reasons for self-harm other than a desire to die. In discussing these reasons for, or functions of, self-harm *it would be wrong to suggest that self-harm is never a symptom of mental illness*. For example, in severe depressive illness a sense of hopelessness and despair can lead to an attempt at suicide that can be seen as a symptom of illness, as can self-harm that is a response to a psychotic delusion.

The so-called non-suicidal reasons for self-harm have been categorized in different ways by different researchers.

One widely quoted approach to thinking about non-suicidal reasons for self-harm adopted a functional approach—which assumes that behaviours are determined by their immediate antecedents and consequences. This behaviourist framework suggests that self-harm is maintained by at least four reinforcement processes (Nock, 2009):

1. Intrapersonal negative reinforcement (here, self-harm decreases or distracts from unwanted thoughts or feelings),
2. Intrapersonal positive reinforcement (where self-harm results in desired pleasant feelings or stimulation),
3. Interpersonal positive reinforcement (here, self-harm results in receiving help or care from others), or
4. Interpersonal negative reinforcement (here, self-harm results in escape from undesired social situations, or where others stop something unpleasant—parents stop fighting, friends stop taunting, and so on).

The most widely studied non-suicidal reasons for self-harm are related to dealing with distress or other unwanted mental states (intrapersonal reasons) and exerting interpersonal influence, including seeking help (interpersonal reasons).

A different approach starts with first-hand accounts from people interviewed about their own self-harm. As shown in Table 3.2, a recent synthesis of research findings using this approach suggests additional personal reasons such as self-validation and self-harm to achieve a personal sense of mastery—which indicate that individuals think there are positive or adaptive functions of self-harm not based only on the social effects of self-harm (Edmondson et al., 2016; Bryant et al., 2021).

Building on this approach using a research technique called Q Methodology, researchers suggested four main functions for non-suicidal self-harm:

- managing unpleasant emotions, thoughts or memories;
- responding in a non-adaptive way to unpleasant emotions, thoughts or memories;
- communicating distress to others;
- obtaining positive feelings or self-appraisals from the act.

CHAPTER 3

Table 3.2 Commonly reported non-suicidal reasons for self-harm. Excluded are psychotic explanations and rarer motives such as self-harm as a political statement or sadomasochistic sexual practice (source data from: Edmondson et al., 2016)

Responding to distress	Self-harm as a positive experience
• Managing distress—managing painful unpleasant emotional states including making emotional pain physical; blocking memories. • Interpersonal influence—changing or responding to how others think or feel; help-seeking. • Punishment—usually of self, occasionally of or by others. • Managing dissociation—that is, either switching off or bringing on feelings of numbness and unreality. • Averting suicide—non-fatal self-harm to ward off suicidal acts or thoughts.	• Gratification—self-harm as comforting or enjoyable. • Sensation seeking—through a sense of non-sexual excitement or arousal. • Experimenting—trying something new. • Protection—of self or others. • Developing a sense of personal mastery. **Defining Self** • Defining boundaries—self-injury is a means of defining personal boundaries. • Responding to sexuality—through self-harm as creating sexual feelings or by expressing sexuality in a symbolic way. • Validation—demonstrating to self and occasionally to others one's strength or the degree of one's suffering. • Self as belonging or fitting in—to a group or subculture. • Having a personal language—including one for remembrance: a means of conjuring up or acknowledging past feelings or memories.

The systematic review by Edmondson and colleagues (2016) and the recent study by Bryant and colleagues (2021) have found that one reason people report for self-harm is that it helps to avert acting on suicidal thinking. In other words, self-harm serves as a strategy for controlling suicidal thoughts and preventing suicide attempt. This offers an explanation for the apparently unusual finding that people who engage in what has been called non-suicidal self-injury are *more* at risk of eventual suicide than are those whose self-harm is identified as having an element of suicidal intent at the time.

It is important to repeat that these reasons are not mutually exclusive. Any one act of self-harm can be explained by more than one reason, and the reasons that a person gives for repeated acts of self-harm can change over time.

Before ending the discussion about the reasons that people report for engaging in self-harm, it is important to draw attention to two common misunderstandings.

First, there is a popular idea that self-harm, particularly, among young people, is 'manipulative' or 'attention-seeking'. This is a dismissive and unhelpful idea that indicates prejudice, stigma, and lack of understanding about self-harm. The primary focus of self-harm is on reducing distress and relieving tension rather than on manipulating other people. At the onset, some people engage in self-harm as a way of signalling their distress to others; however, most people who engage in self-harm repeatedly do so not with the intent to manipulate or seek attention. Remember—if a person engages in self-harm in order to gain another person's attention, then the person who self-harms clearly needs that attention!

The majority of people who engage in self-harm go to some lengths to conceal their self-harming acts, including their bruises, cuts, burns, or scars. People often hide, rather than draw attention to, their self-harm because they are unable to gauge other people's reactions—they may be worried, afraid, or ashamed about other people's reactions, which can be condemnatory and stigmatizing. In fact, this sense of stigma and shame prevents many people who engage in self-harm from seeking help, whether from friends and loved ones or professionals. The strong stigma and condemnatory attitudes that surround self-harm remain a critical challenge to the prevention, intervention, and management of self-harm (Chapters 4 and 5 of this volume discuss self-harm prevention and intervention). It is worth remembering that even though self-harm may not be visibly attention-seeking, concealed self-harm is still a sign that there are underlying tension and distress that warrant attention from persons who are in a position to offer some help—parents, siblings, teachers and other school staff, and other professionals who are in regular contact with young people.

The second common misunderstanding is that the motivation or intention of self-harm can be assumed based on the method of self-harm used. Especially prevalent is the idea that self-injury is an indication that the episode of self-harm is not associated with suicide risk. So-called non-suicidal self-harm is associated with a substantial elevated risk of hospital re-admission and 2 to 5-fold increased risk of subsequent suicide using the same or similar method (Birtwistle et al., 2017).

As an aside, it is worth noting that even though the relationship between self-harm method and suicide intention is unclear and inconsistent, knowing the self-harm method is useful in assessment. For example, cutting is likely to point to a desire to inflict pain, or to see blood flow, or to cause scarring, while taking an overdose is often associated with a desire to sleep or seek oblivion. It can be useful to explore the meaning of these desires.

Knowing what methods people use to self-harm may also be useful in developing strategies to prevent self-harm—whether in the clinic, workplace, school, prison, household, or within the general community context. For example, if self-harm is used to stop the person acting on suicidal thoughts, it has implications for a discussion about restricting access to the means that the person uses to self-harm. A decision by significant others to remove or block access to means of self-harm must be thought through carefully, with the provision of replacement options for positive coping mechanisms.

CHAPTER 3

Putting it all together: the formulation

So far, this chapter has considered the personal and social risks that are most often associated with self-harm, and the reasons for which an individual might undertake an act of self-harm. The most useful way to use any information gathered under these headings is to put it all together (formulate it) into a meaningful account of the episode. This involves asking three main questions, the aim of which can be readily seen from the table that appears at the start of this chapter:

… Were there stressful experiences leading up to the act of self-harm?

In other words—what events, difficulties, or life changes preceded the episode? And what was the meaning of these experiences for the individual? To answer the latter question, it is important to know not just about recent change but about the features of the individual's day-to-day life, what we called problematic current circumstances and membership in at risk groups (see Table 3.1). It is these longer-term circumstances that help explain why a particular recent event comes to be experienced as stressful.

… How could the episode of self-harm be seen as a meaningful response to these circumstances?

The aim here is to move beyond simply seeing self-harm as a symptom of distress, as if it were like crying when we are sad. It is an intentional act with some purpose behind it, however vaguely or uncertainly the individual was thinking about that purpose at the time or can explain it afterwards.

… What individual characteristics help explain why self-harm (as opposed to some other response) was the end result of this set of circumstances?

However stressful life becomes, not everybody (in fact, only a minority) responds with self-harm. So, what are the particular characteristics of the individual that help to explain their actions? While the first two questions can be answered by sensitive questioning of the individual and (sometimes) another person close to them, answers to the third question typically require some interpretation from a third party. For example, it may require some careful probing to identify a long-standing picture of impulsive behaviour, or alcohol misuse, or difficulty with working consistently to solve problems, and then seeing how those characteristics fit into the story about recent self-harm.

The aim of making a formulation like this is to establish a picture of self-harm as a meaningful response to stressful circumstances, rather than simply as a symptom of mental illness or an abnormal personality. Indeed, even when mental illness is present a particular episode of self-harm is likely to be related to personal or social circumstances—for example, poverty that arises from the unemployment so often associated with long-term illness, family tensions associated with (say) an eating disorder.

Seeing the bigger picture: social explanations for self-harm

The primary focus of this book is on the individual. It is however impossible to discuss the reasons for self-harm without noting that there must be social explanations as well. The epidemiology of self-harm has changed dramatically in recent years—involving many more (especially young) people, apparently starting at a younger age, appearing as a significant public health problem in low- and middle-income countries where it is approaching levels seen previously only in developed countries such as those of Western Europe. It has become a culturally understood way of expressing and responding to distress in a way that would have been inconceivable a couple of generations ago. It is beyond the scope of this book to explore the reasons for that, but it serves as a reminder to be careful not to overemphasize the likelihood of individual abnormality in a world where so many social influences affect the presentation of self-harm.

The longer-term outlook after an episode of self-harm

Sometimes problems improve after an episode of self-harm; perhaps the self-harm was a response to a short-lived crisis that has resolved, or perhaps the individual has found ways to tackle their difficulties without further self-harm. It may be that close others (family, friends) have been alerted to the individual's distress and have rallied round to help. In these cases, there may be no longer-term difficulties beyond the immediate unpleasant episode.

As discussed earlier, for some people who repeatedly engage in self-harm the act could be a means to (re)gaining a sense of control or personal strength, or a sense of pleasure. Self-harm could result in achieving a sense of meaningfulness and belonging (with others in a group or subculture). For others the behaviour helps to relief tension and facilitates communication of emotional pain to significant others. These benefits are usually short-lived however, and difficulties are likely to persist or re-emerge later.

The most obvious negatives come from physical effects of the act of self-harm, which may include organ damage from taking medication or scarring from self-injury. Physical treatment may be unpleasant and it has financial consequences for the healthcare system and perhaps the family. Apart from the medical effects, some people report psychological and social consequences including increased feelings of guilt, shame, and poor self-esteem after self-harm, while others experience stigma and its attendant social ostracism and isolation, and poor interpersonal relationships. Especially in low- and middle-income countries, where self-harm is often equated to attempted suicide, survivors of self-harm and their families and loved ones are stigmatized when the self-harm becomes public knowledge.

When the problems associated with self-harm do not resolve other poor outcomes are possible. People with a history of self-harm are more likely to experience educational difficulties, unemployment, and longer-term unhappiness and relationship difficulties.

Repetition—non-fatal and fatal (suicide)

Unsurprisingly, given how frequent longer-term problems are, a history of self-harm is associated with an increased risk for future self-harm. This is especially true for those whose self-harm led to hospital admission. Repetition is especially likely in the first 12 months following an episode of self-harm, when in some studies a third or more of those seen once may repeat the act (Hawton, Bergen, et al., 2015; Castellví et al., 2017). Repetition seems higher in developed countries, and it is important to remember that the majority of people, even in developed countries, do not repeat the act even over several years of follow up.

Suicide is many times commoner (up to 50 times commoner) in the year after a health service contact for self-harm than it is in the general population. Unlike repeated self-harm the risk of suicide is not all front-loaded into the first year after self-harm—estimates suggest that over five years after an act of self-harm about 5% of people will die by suicide. Looked at the other way round, more than half of all those who die by suicide have a previous history of self-harm. A major challenge for suicide prevention is that risks for suicide in this situation are almost identical to the risks associated with non-fatal self-harm, as listed in Table 3.2. The main differences to note are:

Gender—suicide is commoner in men than in women in all countries where it has been studied

Age—the predominance of younger people seen in self-harm is not seen in suicide, and older adults seen after self-harm should be regarded as being at high risk of suicide until proved otherwise

Severe mental illness—bipolar illness in particular is a major risk factor for suicide

Method of self-harm—is not in itself a good pointer to suicide risk, although methods of high potential lethality should be regarded as important risks.

More generally, the best guide is likely to reside in persistence and severity of risks noted in Table 3.1, especially when they are associated with high levels of hopelessness, social isolation, and preoccupation with suicidal ideas.

In summary

- Other than a desire to die, there is a substantial number of reasons for self-harm.
- For some people, self-harm is a way to avert suicide.
- Previous self-harm represents a critical risk factor for repeated self-harm or death by suicide.
- The risk and protective factors for self-harm may be different for young people and adults.

REFERENCES

Birtwistle, J., Kelley, R., House, A., & Owens, D. (2017). Combination of self-harm methods and fatal and non-fatal repetition: a cohort study. *Journal of Affective Disorders*, *218*, 188–194. https://doi.org/10.1016/j.jad.2017.04.027

Bryant, L. D., O'Shea, R., Farley, K., Brennan, C., Crosby, H. F., Guthrie, E., & House, A. (2021). Understanding the functions of repeated self-harm: a Q methodology approach. *Social Science & Medicine*, *268*, 113527. https://doi.org/10.1016/j.socsci med.2020.113527

Castellví, P., Lucas-Romero, E., Miranda-Mendizábal, A., Parés-Badell, O., Almenara, J., Alonso, I., Blasco, M., Cebrià, A., Gabilondo, A., & Gili, M. (2017). Longitudinal association between self-injurious thoughts and behaviors and suicidal behavior in adolescents and young adults: a systematic review with meta-analysis. *Journal of Affective Disorders*, *215*, 37–48. https://doi.org/10.1016/j.jad.2017.03.035

Edmondson, A. J., Brennan, C. A., & House, A. O. (2016). Non-suicidal reasons for self-harm: a systematic review of self-reported accounts. *Journal of Affective Disorders*, *191*, 109–117. https://doi.org/10.1016/j.jad.2015.11.043

Hawton, K., Bergen, H., Cooper, J., Turnbull, P., Waters, K., Ness, J., & Kapur, N. (2015). Suicide following self-harm: findings from the multicentre study of self-harm in England, 2000–2012. *Journal of Affective Disorders*, *175*, 147–151. https://doi.org/10.1016/ j.jad.2014.12.062

Nock, M. K. (2009). Why do people hurt themselves? New insights into the nature and functions of self-injury. *Current Directions in Psychological Science*, *18*(2), 78–83. https:// doi.org/10.1111/j.1467-8721.2009.01613.x

Part 2

Intervention for and prevention of self-harm

CHAPTER 4

Self-harm prevention in clinical and non-clinical contexts

KEY POINTS

- The United Nations Sustainable Development Goals direct global attention to self-harm prevention.
- Preventing self-harm is important because self-harm is the strongest known risk for suicide.
- Several population-level prevention programmes suggest the possibility of reducing self-harm.
- Responsible media reporting and portrayal of self-harm can contribute to prevent self-harm, particularly in young people.
- Effective restriction and banning of access to highly lethal and hazardous means of self-harm is part of a wider suicide prevention strategy: they require legislation and political will.

Self-harm is now recognized as a global public health problem, and the development of preventive strategies and assessment of their effectiveness continues to engage the attention of researchers, interventionists, and policymakers. Notably, indicator 3·4·2 of the United Nations Sustainable Development Goals seeks to reduce premature mortality from suicide by one-third by the year 2030. Considering that self-harm is the biggest risk for suicide across all age groups, this target of the Sustainable Development Goals directs global attention to self-harm prevention.

Broadly, self-harm prevention can be at the individual level or population level.

Individual-level prevention approaches typically involve assessment and intervention for self-harm in groups identified as being at high risk, such as those with known mental health problems (for primary prevention) or those who have already reported episode(s) of self-harm (for secondary prevention). Such secondary preventive activities are often conducted at clinical services and involve asking people about their experience of self-harm thoughts, particularly if they are presenting with anxiety, depression, thoughts of hopelessness, low self-esteem, or other negative emotions or undesirable thoughts. Contrary to popular belief, studies have shown that asking people about their self-harm ideas and thoughts does not heighten the risk of self-harm occurring, rather—along with other benefits, it can lead to improvement in mood (DeCou & Schumann, 2018). Specific individual-level preventive measures and interventions are covered in Chapter 5.

Population-level approaches to self-harm prevention are typically aimed at decreasing the incidence of self-harm by reducing or eliminating the risk factors and enhancing the protective factors in the whole population or an identifiable group or specific places such as schools, workplaces, or places of worship. Population-based prevention strategies are now viewed as important, given that most people (especially young people) who self-harm do not present to clinical care at the time, and indeed the majority of people who self-harm are unknown to clinical services at all. As indicated in the preceding chapter, this low level of presenting for professional care is driven in part by the stigma associated with self-harm and, in some contexts, the criminal status of the behaviour. It is worthy of note that thus far most of what we know about the effectiveness of prevention and intervention comes from research conducted in high-income countries. We know less than enough from low- and middle-income contexts about what works in self-harm prevention.

Whole population interventions

Primary prevention programmes may include one or more components (Box 4.1).

Education and awareness-raising aims to improve general understanding of states of distress like depression and anxiety—what the symptoms can be, how to recognize them in oneself or others, to understand how common they are and not something to be ashamed of or to criticize. Self-harm is explained as a common response to distress, especially in young people.

Skills training typically involves outlining the basic elements of problem-solving, of thinking about how to respond to stressful events so that they can be made less stressful, or coped with if they cannot be altered.

Encouraging help-seeking is partly a way to challenge attitudes by saying—you are not alone with this—and partly an opportunity to provide information on the types of help available, which can vary considerably from place to place.

Fostering support networks aims to reduce the sense of isolation and loneliness that can affect the mental health of so many people. It may involve encouraging the individual to use their (new!) problem-solving skills to reconnect with people they have been avoiding, or it may involve introducing the individual to

---

Box 4.1 Primary prevention of self-harm: some typical components

- Education and awareness-raising;
- Skills training;
- Encouraging help-seeking;
- Fostering support networks;
- Improving the local environment—for example, in school or work.

---

new networks through, for example, contact with third-sector (voluntary or non-official) organizations or community groups. An advantage of widening social networks is that it can introduce new people who may be a source of helpful advice and information about how to tackle current problems.

Improving the local environment depends upon the prevention programme building relationships with other organizations. For example, it might be important to help schools that are trying to implement an anti-bullying programme or work with a local employer to encourage supporting practice in relation to time off work with mental health problems.

One illustrative example is the Youth Aware of Mental Health Programme, which targeted pupils aged 14–16 years old recruited from 168 schools across 10 European Union countries (Wasserman et al., 2015). Besides awareness-raising about risks and protective factors for youth self-harm and suicide, the programme also involves literacy about depression and anxiety and strategies for improving young people's skills to deal with life adversities, distress, and self-harming behaviours. It was delivered through workshops accompanied by an explanatory booklet, lectures about mental health topics, and posters in schools. Evaluation in a randomized trial showed that it reduced rates of self-harm and also reduced the more severe thoughts about self-harm and suicide.

Restriction of access to means of self-harm involves limiting access to potentially dangerous objects, high-frequency locations, and toxic substances that are used as means of self-harm. Apart from making potentially lethal means of self-harm unavailable, restricting access to means of self-harm also contributes to buying time during which the strength of self-harm thoughts may reduce. Relatedly, if access to a highly dangerous self-harm method has been restricted and the person experiencing a self-harm crisis is unable to defer their self-harm, they frequently use less dangerous methods.

Restricting the number of capsules or tablets of prescription medicines and limiting the pack sizes of over-the-counter medicines such as paracetamol and other medicines that are commonly used for self-poisoning have contributed to the reduction in intentional overdose and self-poisoning with these medicines in Australia and the UK. In lower-income and predominantly rural settings, regulations governing the sale of pesticides are important. Such measures are not currently possible in every country. There is concern, however, about whether the result is simply the substitution of a different method, which may itself be dangerous.

Despite their usefulness, these restrictions and bans can seem intrusive to some community members. Hence, it is worth emphasizing that the introduction and enforcement of such public health initiatives to limit or ban access to means of self-harm require legislation and political will.

Alcohol and drug policy can have an effect on self-harm as a secondary benefit. Alcohol consumption is extremely common in the hours before an act of self-harm, so much so that it may be thought of as a part of the build-up to the act. It may be that drinking too much is part of a self-poisoning episode, or alcohol may have an effect by exacerbating low mood or by encouraging impulsivity. And unhealthy use of illicit substances is both a risk for self-harm and a means of intentional self-harm.

As mentioned in Chapter 3, some caution must be exercised when restricting access to the means that people use to self-harm, as acts of self-harm represent a means to avert suicide, particularly in some young people. There must be provision of replacement options for positive coping mechanisms (some helpful approaches are discussed in Chapter 5).

Social media can be a resource although they are often discussed for their potentially harmful effects, and it can be easy to forget that they may be a useful source of support or information for those at risk of self-harm.

There is evidence that the *creation and sharing of self-harm-related content* online can contribute to reducing self-harm urges by providing alternative outlets for difficult emotions.

Other studies have specifically explored self-harm and suicide-related media portrayals focused on *messages of hope, mastery over a crisis, or (continuous) recovery*. Persons exposed to such positive media portrayal have reported experiencing a decrease in self-harm urges, suicidal ideation, reduced feelings of distress, and increased hope.

The internet or social media has also been found to afford isolated or lonely individuals, who might not present to professional care, *a sense of belonging and support*. This is especially important given what we know about how many people hide their feelings, find it difficult to confide in those around them, and are ashamed of feelings of depression or thoughts about suicide or self-harm.

Social media can be used actively to achieve some of these benefits and there are a number of professionally run sites along those lines (see for example self-injury outreach www.sioutreach.org). A particularly impressive development is the #chatsafe programme, which was co-developed by professionals and young people. The #chatsafe project provides complementary guidelines, co-produced with young people designed to facilitate supportive and safe peer-peer communication on social media about self-harm and suicide among young people. Thus, the programme's site offers advice on topics such as how to share thoughts and feelings online and how to communicate with others affected by suicide. The recent globalization of the #chatsafe guidelines (www.orygen.org.au/chatsafe)—originally developed in Australia—is also beginning to receive positive evaluative reports.

Targeted interventions

School-based programmes
Some successful whole-school programmes include screening at-risk school-going young people, awareness-raising and psychological skills training, and gatekeeper training. Evidence from high-income countries suggests that screening programmes help school professionals identify and recognize students who are at risk

of self-harm and facilitate referrals for professional mental healthcare to address untreated mental health problems. However, besides the likelihood of one-time screening yielding false negatives, school-based screening programmes can also involve high costs for schools, including those associated with high levels of false positives that lead to unnecessary further assessment, distress, and unwarranted intervention. For these reasons, school-based screening is not recommended by the US Preventive Services Taskforce.

A particular risk for self-harm among school-age young people comes from peer pressure and bullying (Heerde & Hemphill, 2019). Perhaps surprisingly, it is not just being a victim of bullying that is important but also being a perpetrator. School-based programmes aimed at reducing bullying and supporting those involved in it are important in their own right, and because a reduction in bullying is one route to reducing self-harm.

Training may be organized in schools, health facilities, or the community. It involves training adults (such as school staff, opinion leaders, community leaders, and healthcare professionals) and young people (including peers and siblings) to be able to recognize risks and warning signs of self-harm and refer or facilitate contact with appropriate professional support sources. Again, however, the risk of false positives is high, and, in that light it is better to consider other options: there is evidence to suggest that gatekeeper training improves knowledge and supportive attitudes about self-harm, can decrease self-harm and improve help-seeking. While more evidence is needed, whole-school training approaches also have the potential to improve school culture, climate, and ethos regarding the mental well-being of students.

Prisons and other custodial settings

Peer-support programmes, particularly peer-led problem-solving therapy, have been found to lead to significant reductions in self-harm episodes. In this approach, prisoners are trained in problem-solving skills and become peer-support mentors across the intervention period. Recent evidence from an English prison suggests that prisoners who receive problem-solving skills training from peer mentors at least once report reduced episodes of self-harm following the intervention (Perry et al., 2021).

Studies have consistently shown a relationship between self-harm and aggression; approaches to anger management may be valuable for the effect they have on prison life and, related to improved alternative approaches to stress, may help to reduce self-harm.

Media policy

Mainstream media

The global literature is replete with concerns that inappropriate reporting and portrayal of self-harm in mainstream media is associated with an increased risk of self-harm, as it normalizes self-harm, triggers self-harm urges, or leads to increased depression. In particular, media contents which include dramatic and detailed reporting and portrayal of self-harm methods have been suggested to contribute significantly to self-harm in young people. For example, the available findings from recent research studying the effects of Netflix's TV series '13 Reasons Why' Season 1 released globally in Spring 2017 suggested a link between the TV series and increases in self-harm, particularly in young people.

The development and application of guidelines on reporting and portrayal of self-harm and suicide in the media have been found as a useful prevention and intervention strategy. These recommended media guidelines have been developed by the WHO, leading experts in self-harm and suicide prevention, several key public health organizations, schools of journalism and key journalists, media organizations, and in collaboration with internet safety experts.

Social media

An important differentiating feature of social media is that their content is generated by users themselves and therefore not subject to guidelines in the same way as mainstream media. There are concerns that self-harm content in social media is harmful through the effects of lowering mood or encouraging or glamorizing self-harm. These concerns have been brought to the fore by a high-profile case in the UK in which the suicide of a young girl was attributed in part to exposure to such material—an exposure exacerbated by algorithms that suggested continuing online searches for depression and self-harm content with recommendations to further postings. Legislation designed to impose a duty on tech companies to maintain safety on all their online platforms is being considered in a number of countries, although there are likely to be considerable difficulties in defining what exactly constitutes safe or harmful exposure.

Self-harm prevention as a secondary benefit of other programmes

There are a number of groups in society whose members are at increased risk of self-harm, but where their primary needs are in other spheres—for better access to general medical or mental health services, to education or vocational training to improve employment prospects, or to better social support and protection against stigmatization or discrimination in day-to-day life. It may be that in meeting these primary needs, there is a reduction in self-harm as a result of any improvement made.

Examples include:

- people with learning disability or autism
- people who are LGBTQ+
- street-connected people

- young people not in education, employment, or training
- no stable family support—including young people leaving the care system, the isolated elderly adult.

Mental health promotion

Mental health promotion relates to enhancing individuals' and communities' capacity to master and increase control over their lives and improve their mental health. Over the years, civil society organizations, social care professionals, community-based organizations, third-sector organizations and related organizations around the world—for example, Samaritans, MIND, International Association for Suicide Prevention [IASP], Harmless, Befrienders International, and LifeLine International [LLI]—have been known to have direct and significant contact with people who may be at risk of self-harm, suicide, or mental health problems. They make important contributions towards improving mental health and supporting self-harm and suicide prevention among individuals and communities. Although many of these organizations were formed to operate in their Western countries of origin, today, several of them (IASP, LLI, Befrienders International) are reaching out and extending support to self-harm and suicide prevention programmes across several low- and middle-income countries, particularly, in sub-Saharan Africa, South-East Asia, and South America. To contribute to self-harm prevention, typically, efforts by these organizations seek to promote good mental health and well-being, tackle mental health inequalities, discrimination, and stigma, facilitate access to formal care, support people in crisis or distress (through toll-free helpline and referral services), and promote resilience and recovery among vulnerable groups and populations.

Young people's and adults' suggestions for self-harm prevention

So far what has been described in this book is based almost entirely upon initiatives by professionals. However, the accounts and perspectives of people with personal experience can also show what psychosocial and health support should look like, how it can contribute to recovery, and how such support could mean different things to different people. There is now a growing interest in considering people with personal experience as stakeholders in mental health service provision and critical agents of change towards improving public awareness of mental health and the integration and acceptance of people experiencing mental health problems (WHO, 2022). Their participation is key to improving mental healthcare and outcomes. Thus, it is recognized that the integration of the perspectives of people with personal experience in self-harm intervention and prevention efforts can lead to not only the empowerment of patients but also contribute to improving the responses and learnings of healthcare professionals.

Some recent studies have explored and synthesized first-hand accounts of people with personal experience about what they think is helpful towards reducing or stopping self-harm. The complex and multicausal nature of self-harm also presupposes that the suggestions by people with personal experience of self-harm for prevention would be multipronged in form, relating to several areas or domains of personal life, interpersonal relationships, and the broader social circumstances within which they live. Also, considering that self-harm is culture- and context-driven, preventive measures suggested by a person or a group of people in a given culture or context may not necessarily apply to another person or group of people in the same or different context. Thus, whereas suggestions for self-harm prevention may be potentially informative for universal prevention efforts, they may require further adaptation to suit targeted preventive programmes.

A recent systematic synthesis of the global evidence by a team of researchers from the UK with a longstanding interest in self-harm prevention (Brennan et al., 2023) has highlighted some first-hand accounts and suggestions. For example, replacement of acts of self-harm with more positive experiences such as acts of self-care; reflective thinking about the determinants of self-harm; managing provocations through recognizing and avoiding the situations that present as triggers of self-harm; awareness of contributing factors such as drinking alcohol. The review also noted the importance of seeking to establish lasting changes in social relationships and interpersonal circumstances, and not just focusing on changing feelings about oneself. Among adults, the importance of lasting structural changes in circumstances was highlighted. For example, leaving toxic relationships, finding purpose through employment, or moving out of one's family home.

Recent research among young people with personal experience of self-harm in low- and middle-income countries has highlighted suggestions ranging from microsystem changes such as changing restrictive and punitive patriarchal parenting styles (encouraging parents and caregivers to adopt supportive parenting styles that emphasize open parent–child communication) to macrosystem level changes, including formulating and implementing (both existing and new) conventions, laws and policies protecting young people, creating pro-mental health school environments, and improving the economic circumstances of families and communities through concerted pursuit of poverty reduction policies by governments.

In summary

- Even though some social media contents can have potentially harmful effects, the creation and sharing of self-harm-related content online can also contribute to reducing self-harm urges by providing alternative outlets for difficult emotions.
- Whole-school preventive approaches have the potential to improve school culture, climate, and ethos regarding mental well-being of students.
- Peer-led problem-solving therapy skills intervention has been found to lead to significant reductions in self-harm episodes in prisoners.
- The integration of the perspectives of people with personal experience in self-harm intervention and prevention efforts can lead to patient empowerment and improved empathic responses and learnings of healthcare professionals.

REFERENCES

Brennan, C. A., Crosby, H., Sass, C., Farley, K. L., Bryant, L. D., Rodriquez-Lopez, R., Romeu, D., Mitchell, E., House, A. O., & Guthrie, E. (2023). What helps people to reduce or stop self-harm? A systematic review and meta-synthesis of first-hand accounts. *Journal of Public Health*, *45*(1), 154–161. https://doi.org/10.1093/pubmed/fdac022

DeCou, C. R., & Schumann, M. E. (2018). On the iatrogenic risk of assessing suicidality: a meta-analysis. *Suicide and Life-Threatening Behavior*, *48*(5), 531–543. https://doi.org/10.1111/sltb.12368

Heerde, J. A., & Hemphill, S. A. (2019). Are bullying perpetration and victimization associated with adolescent deliberate self-harm? A meta-analysis. *Archives of Suicide Research*, *23*(3), 353–381. https://doi.org/10.1080/13811118.2018.1472690

Perry, A. E., Waterman, M. G., Dale, V., Moore, K., & House, A. (2021). The effect of a peer-led problem-support mentor intervention on self-harm and violence in prison: an interrupted time series analysis using routinely collected prison data. *EClinicalMedicine*, *32*, 100702. https://doi.org/10.1016/j.eclinm.2020.100702

Wasserman, D., Hoven, C. W., Wasserman, C., Wall, M., Eisenberg, R., Hadlaczky, G., Kelleher, I., Sarchiapone, M., Apter, A., & Balazs, J. (2015). School-based suicide prevention programmes: the SEYLE cluster-randomised, controlled trial. *The Lancet*, *385*(9977), 1536–1544. https://doi.org/10.1016/S0140-6736(14)61213-7

WHO (2022). *World mental health report: transforming mental health for all*. World Health Organization.

Intervention in clinical and non-clinical contexts

KEY POINTS

- The first response when self-harm is presented will be to ensure that any physical harm is properly treated and that any further risk is assessed and treated.
- The emphasis in therapy may vary according to the individual's circumstances.
- Therapy may be a response to self-harm, risked or actual, but it does not need to be entirely focused on self-harm.
- Psychological therapies aim at exploring ways to reduce or remove stresses, or of coping with them if they are not amenable to change.

Individual-level interventions for self-harm

Self-harm can present in different environments—schools and colleges, prisons and other correctional facilities, community services, medical settings. In each of these environments the first response will be to ensure that any physical harm is properly treated—cleaning and caring for wounds, limiting damage from poisoning, and so on. Beyond this physical treatment, any help for the individual is likely to involve talking, either in an informal supportive way or as part of what have been called talking therapies or psychological therapies.

In this chapter we will outline the main features of psychological therapies that may be offered as a response to self-harm. We will also consider how these therapeutic approaches can be modified for use in settings where therapy isn't available, and with groups of people with particular risks or special problems. When we say 'as a response to self-harm' we have two situations in mind: the first involves a person who has recently self-harmed and has either presented for help or their self-harm has come to light in other ways—during a conversation, or because scars have been noticed, for example. The second involves a person who has not self-harmed but is at risk of doing so, because of their current circumstances and thoughts and feelings. The approach in each case is much the same although of course the emphasis may vary according to the individual's circumstances.

The focus of therapy

It is worth saying that intervention may be a response to self-harm, risked or actual, but it does not need to be entirely focused on self-harm. People value therapy that takes account of them as a person with whatever problems or feelings they have; certainly, it helps to see somebody who understands and is interested in self-harm, but they don't want to be approached as if that's the only important thing about them.

Immediate circumstances

As we have seen, for many people there has been some sort of stressful experience immediately before an episode of self-harm. These experiences may be single events—an argument, the break-up of a relationship, unexpected bad news—or they may involve more long-standing difficulties such as debt, bullying or other abuse, or chronic pain. Therapy is aimed at clarifying exactly what these issues are and why they are important, with the aim of exploring ways to reduce or remove these stresses, or of coping with them if they are not amenable to change.

Current emotional state and cognitive state

Self-harm is almost always associated with emotional distress. Such negative feelings come with negative thoughts which themselves are likely to be relevant such as ideas of hopelessness or personal worthlessness. Since these feelings and thoughts often provide the link between personal circumstances and self-harm, therapy is aimed at identifying them and exploring ways to reduce or eliminate them, or at least to find ways of minimizing their impact.

Associated mental disorders

Although most people who self-harm are not mentally ill, for those who are then an aim of therapy can be to treat the mental disorder. Examples include an eating disorder, OCD, or severe and persistent depressive disorder. Psychosis is rare and if it is present then, as with these other mental disorders, specialist mental health assessment and treatment is indicated before attempting therapy for any associated self-harm.

Types of therapy

In this section we review the main types of therapy that have been evaluated in self-harm, outlining their defining features and considering the rationale for using the particular therapeutic approach.

... Very brief (typically a one-off session) approaches

The rationale for very brief interventions is a practical one. Many people will not or cannot come back for further meetings with a therapist or other specialist, or there may be nobody available to provide further help. So the opportunity to offer something helpful has to be taken in the single contact that is taking place here and now.

Therapeutic assessment ± follow-up

Assessment is often discussed as if it just involves gathering information, to help assess risk for example, but it can be therapeutic as well as fact-finding. Sympathetic question about somebody's situation and problems can lead to sharing that in itself brings emotional relief. And explaining problems to another person can lead to new ways of thinking about them and suggest possible solutions that haven't occurred when brooding alone. Often, these one-off sessions are followed up with simple contacts by telephone, text message, or postcard—expressing the hope that things are going well and encouraging help-seeking if problems persist.

Safety planning

Another approach that can be delivered in a single session involves producing a safety plan.

What a safety plan includes is a list of actions somebody can take when they feel so bad that there is a risk of self-harm. It is worth thinking these things through in advance because in the middle of a crisis when somebody is struggling with their feelings and thoughts it can be too difficult to think clearly about what to do that is positive.

A safety plan should not be given to somebody, it should be completed in discussion with them—taking into account what they want to try, what is practical given their circumstances and so on. If it involves contacting other people then it is worth letting those people know in advance if possible and perhaps sharing the plan with them: this is a decision that can only be made by the person whose plan it is.

A typical example of a safety plan is shown in the box. A plan like this can be drawn up by anybody who understands the principle involved and is willing to spend a bit of time working to develop a plan with the person who will use it (Box 5.1).

... Brief (typically 4–6 sessions) approaches

Beyond these single session interventions, the next level of therapy involves a number of sessions, typically one or two weeks apart. The usual number of contacts rarely goes above six because, again, few people can or will attend for more. Sometimes there may be fewer and follow-ups can be arranged by telephone if it is available.

A major challenge to delivering even brief interventions in low-income countries is cost, both in terms of therapy time and cost to the individual (travel, time of work, and so on). There are online or telephone-delivered equivalents, but they are not always feasible and can be a threat to confidentiality. This lack of access to brief therapies is one aspect of global health inequality that can only be tackled by reform of mental health service provision.

Box 5.1 Example of a safety plan	
Safety plan for:	Date:
If I am feeling overwhelmed and in danger of acting on thoughts of self-harm, I will:	
Statement *Write a clear statement using 'I' that you can read and repeat to yourself, e.g. 'I will give myself time to try to take care of myself and help myself feel a bit better.'*	
Someone to call I will call one of the following people: *(It's a good idea to save these numbers in your phone contacts under a relevant heading like 'Help'. You could also see if one or more of the listed people would agree to keep a copy of your safety plan and help talk you through it if necessary)*	Friend: Parent/relative: Support worker: Friend: Other:
Remove dangerous items: *Write down what you can do to make it more difficult for you to harm yourself (e.g. not drinking alcohol while you are feeling this way, not stockpiling medication, removing, or locking away razor blades, knives, rope.)*	I will make myself safe from acting impulsively by ...
Relaxing or soothing activities: *Go for a walk; focus on my breathing; listen to relaxing or uplifting music*	I will choose something from my list of self-soothing activities and focus on it for at least 20 minutes
Write down one or more coping statements that you can repeat to yourself, e.g. 'I have survived so far, and I will make a commitment to surviving for another hour/day.'	I will remind myself of my coping statements and what has helped me before
Write down places you may be able to go if you still feel at risk, e.g. friend who has agreed to be available emergency support services; nearest A&E remembering to tell them you feel you are a danger to yourself	If I still feel suicidal and at risk a safe place, I can go to is ...

Problem-solving therapy

The rationale of problem-solving is straightforward: if self-harm is a response to personal problems, then learning new ways to deal with life problems is likely to reduce the recourse to self-harm. Active problem-solvers are likely to feel more self-confident and able to cope in other ways. In outline, the aim is to explain the

Table 5.1 Problem-solving plan	
Steps in problem-solving	**Completing the step**
Write a problem list	Try to be as specific as possible in defining what the problem is
Choose a problem to tackle	It may be the most important, or the easiest to solve, or the one that needs most immediate attention
List possible solutions to the chosen problem	Again, try to be as specific as possible
Choose the solution you will try first	And think about why that looks like the best to try first
Review how it went	If it was a success, think why—and then pick another problem to tackle, if it didn't work don't give up; think about what went wrong and try again either improving how to use try the solution or choosing a different one

steps of active problem-solving and then to work through the process during sessions. The various steps are outlined in the accompanying text box (Table 5.1).

In practice, this apparently simple intervention can run into difficulties. Some people find it hard to grasp and apply the principles—they jump at the first problem they think of or find it difficult to be specific, they think of one solution and keep trying it without asking themselves why it isn't working, or they give up if the first solution they try isn't immediately effective. For these reasons problem-solving therapy is more likely to be effective if delivered by somebody with practical experience in working with troubled people and with training in the technique and in how to respond to common problems.

Brief focused psychological therapies

There are a number of standardized therapies that focus on specific aspects of a person's life and mental state and which can be delivered in relatively few sessions. They are delivered by a therapist trained in the use of the therapy who (at least in research studies) is likely to have access to a therapy manual detailing the main techniques and giving examples. The three most widely used have been cognitive behavioural therapy (CBT), acceptance and commitment therapy (ACT), and psychodynamic interpersonal therapy (PIT).

In CBT for self-harm treatment usually starts with the assessment of the most recent episode of self-harm (circumstances at the time of the episode, motives and reasons for self-harm, cognitions, emotions, and behaviour prior to and at the time of the episode). The therapist and patient then investigated how emotional, cognitive, and behavioural factors played a part in the self-harm. Specific factors include unhelpful ways of thinking and poor problem-solving. Near the end of therapy relapse prevention can be addressed as well. The treatment is first and foremost an individual one.

In ACT, therapy targets mainly the tendency to avoid unwanted thoughts or emotions. The six core processes of ACT are: acceptance of uncomfortable private experiences (thoughts, feelings, or physical sensations); distancing from one's own uncomfortable thoughts; being present (directing attention to present events and experiences rather than focusing on the past or future); self-awareness in the present moment through the 'observing self;' identification of personal values; and commitment to action in line with the identified values.

In psychodynamic interpersonal therapy, therapy focuses on: the client's emotional life (which is what the term 'psychodynamic' refers to); the client's relationships with other people (which is what the term 'interpersonal' refers to); and how problems with managing feelings and relationships might link with difficult experiences in the client's past, particularly with their parents or other important people. The goal of therapy is for the client to get a better understanding of their difficulties with feelings and relationships, so that they can manage their personal problems more effectively.

Although these therapies can sound as if they are quite different, and each does require its own specific therapist training, in reality they are very similar in effect. This is likely to be because of the non-specific or generalizable therapy effects— the benefits of spending time with somebody warm and interested who spends time trying to understand one's problems, is accepting and non-judgemental and trustworthy in a way that allows a *therapeutic alliance* to develop, and who is competent and can support expectations of improvement. These non-specific components of effective therapies, as identified by researchers, are similar to the features of therapy valued by recipients of therapy, which are therefore important in patient-centred care (see Chapter 7).

... More extensive therapies (may be 6–12 months)

Dialectical behaviour therapy (DBT) is a modification of CBT with four components: mindfulness; distress tolerance; emotion regulation; interpersonal effectiveness. It is delivered 1:1 and in group format for up to 12 months. Therapists require specialist training, and the therapy is intensive and therefore expensive to deliver. The justification is that it has been developed to help people who repeatedly self-harm in the setting of other personal problems, such as difficulty in establishing and maintaining intimate trusting relationships, and a tendency to rapid and at times unpredictable mood changes that are distinguishable from the mood swings of bipolar illness by virtue of being relatively short-lived.

Psychodynamic or psychoanalytic therapies are not readily available in many countries, because of lack of suitable trained therapists and because they have rarely been seen as having the necessary flexibility in application to suit the target population. However, a recent review (Briggs et al., 2019) suggests that when they have been used they produce results similar to those of other therapies as judged by reductions in rates of subsequent episodes.

Interventions in special settings

School-based therapies

Because self-harm is so common in young people, most of whom go to school, there is a question of whether school-based intervention is effective (Cox & Hetrick, 2017). It seems that in principle it may be, but in many instances the practicalities of therapy deliver do not make this a feasible option. Alternatives such as school-based counselling or support are more practical in most settings, although there is little research by which to judge their effectiveness.

Apart from practicalities, another challenge for school-based therapy is concerns about confidentiality. Digital interventions (Stefanopoulou et al., 2020) have become popular partly for this reason, and partly because time spent online is so widespread among young people. There are two main variants. One is that mobile phones, tablets, or laptops can be used as a platform for the delivery of therapies such as CBT that have been modified for digital delivery. This approach can be cumbersome and doesn't necessarily reflect how young people engage with the online world, in ways that are more interactive and using different media. In Chapter 6 we review some ways in which social media and other online resources are being used to help young people.

Interventions in prisons, youth offender, and other correctional facilities

Therapy in custodial settings has its own challenges. Separation of inmates from social support and opportunities for problem-solving means that it is difficult to benefit from advances made in the artificial environment of therapy by application in the more natural social world. And custodial settings are often themselves adverse environments, with bullying and the constant threat of violence likely to be counter-therapeutic.

Studies conducted in prisons, community-based forensic settings, forensic hospital settings, and other custodial contexts have shown varying levels of impact of different therapies and models of care on self-harm and risk of self-harm relative to treatment as usual:

- Group-based treatment programmes: This involves mainly cognitive behavioural suicide prevention therapy—a structured, time-bound psychosocial intervention developed to treat individuals experiencing suicidal thinking or self-harm. It is typically modularized into a few components (attention broadening, cognitive restructuring, mood management and behavioural activation, problem-solving training, and improving self-esteem and positive schema). Typically, the delivery of the programme consists of weekly several sessions of up to 1 hour per session.

Research has not clearly established the impact of tailored programmes or individual treatment models (such as dialectical behavioural therapy, psychodynamic interpersonal therapy), and changes in policy and legislation (such as changes to administrative policies and clinical procedures, criminal law reforms, and environmental modifications) on self-harm in prison and detention contexts. However, cognitive restructuring, social skills, self-harm screening practices, and problem-solving skills training have been found to show potential in reducing self-harm and suicide among young people in detention (Carter et al., 2022).

Interventions for high-risk groups

Sexual and gender minority

Persons identifying as sexual and gender minorities are at an elevated risk of self-harm, but sexual and gender minority people may face double jeopardy in countries where their sexual and gender status is illegal and so is self-harm and suicide. Many societies have made progress in accepting the sexual and gender minority population, but the challenges of self-harm and suicide among sexual and gender minority youth in particular suggests there is still much to be done. It is now well established that negative family attitudes, alienation and rejection, and bullying at school when young people 'come out' increase the risk of self-harm.

School and family support may be critical to reducing self-harm among sexual and gender minority youth. Anti-bullying policies can contribute to supportive school climate and sense of belonging. Enforcing non-discriminatory clauses in the healthcare system can also potentially promote equity and professional (mental) health seeking among this population.

Individual-level interventions focused on sexual and gender minority-affirming values and principles can effectively reduce mental distress and self-stigma. Specifically, interventions drawing on the principles of CBT targeting minority-related stressors can be effective at reducing depression, anxiety, internalized stigma, alcohol use among sexual and gender minority youth. Considering the connection between depression, anxiety, internalized stigma, and self-harm, these interventions may also be effective for reducing self-harm in sexual and gender minority youth.

While studies are still needed to test the long-term contributions of interpersonal-level interventions to reducing discrimination and self-harm among sexual and gender minority youth, there is evidence to suggest that attachment-based family therapy can decrease thoughts of self-harm in this population. Typically, interpersonal-level interventions targeting parents of sexual and gender minority youth include showing educational films, interactive online modules, and expressive writing. Most of these interpersonal-level interventions seek to increase contact and empathy with sexual and gender minority people; teach caregivers, teachers, healthcare providers, and peers to reduce discrimination against persons identifying as sexual and gender minority; and increase sexual and gender minority-affirming principles and behaviours.

Severe physical illness, pain, and disability

Psychotherapeutic approaches to physical illness may have benefits in a number of areas that are relevant to reducing self-harm:

- Increasing a sense of personal control and self-efficacy—an example is the use of motivational interviewing to facilitate greater social and physical rehabilitation;
- Treatment of associated depression;
- Improvement of interpersonal function, especially when avoidance is a significant component of disability;
- Reducing overuse of medication, such as potent analgesia for chronic pain, that can impair quality of life and lower mood without controlling pain adequately.

Learning disability and autism

Until recently, the main approach for this population has been strongly influenced by approaches derived from behaviour therapy.

As a first step, caregivers can maintain a journal to monitor and track instances of self-harm, including recording where it occurred, what was happening, who was present, what occurred immediately before and after the episode. For example, how did other people respond, did the child get to avoid or escape or leave or delay a difficult situation? It is helpful to have written records as they provide details that may otherwise go unnoticed and they are more reliable than random recollections which may be emotionally charged.

A functional behavioural assessment can be helpful in this regard. Professionals, including teachers and clinicians, can help families or parents to identify the functions of the self-harming behaviour for the individual. Often the outcome of an assessment is a behaviour intervention plan that serves to guide parents and teachers to teach and reward desirable, positive behaviours in persons who self-harm. Typically, such a plan includes:

i.   Defining the behaviour: using specific, observable language to describe what the self-harm may look like and the form it can take.

ii. Gathering and analysing information: exploring where, how, and when the behaviour is occurring, the effects of the behaviour, and the people and situations that seem to be related.

iii. Identifying motivations or reasons: making an informed guess regarding what might be causing the self-harm or what the child may be attempting to convey or communicate.

iv. Making a plan to address the situation: identifying the specific helpful responses, actions, and interventions towards improving communication or reducing triggers of the self-harm.

The literature identifies two main intervention options once the antecedent factors or events reinforcing the self-harm have been identified (Edelson et al., 2016).

The first is non-contingent reinforcement, a short-term intervention option to reduce self-harm by providing the person with the reinforcer maintaining self-harm on a schedule largely separate from the occurrence of the behaviour. Non-contingent reinforcement leads to decreases in the influence of the reinforcer that is maintaining the self-harm by reducing its motivational value and disrupting the connection between engaging in self-harm and obtaining access to the event at the same time.

The second treatment option for reinforcement-maintained self-harm is functional communication training which aims to teach and encourage the person to use communicative behaviours that serve the same function as the self-harm. This approach can be effective in decreasing self-harm maintained by socially mediated outcomes such as obtaining access to preferred items (such as toys) or activities, social interaction, and being enabled to move out of uncomfortable situations. Talking therapies need modification (reasonable adjustments); different emotional vocabulary, more time; often less control over immediate conditions. Experts have recommended that developing individualized approaches to manage these difficulties, and a combination of both interventions can produce meaningful reductions of self-harm.

More recently it has become clear that other sorts of psychological therapy may be possible, especially for those with less severe disability, provided the therapy is modified to meet the needs of the population (see for example Jahoda et al., 2018).

Targeting services in low-resource settings

Most of what we know through published research about individual-level therapies and interventions comes from high-income countries; not much is known from low- and middle-income countries, mainly due to their problems with shortage and unavailability of trained specialists and professionals. It is also worth remembering that many people with mental illness in low- and middle-income countries do not receive the needed professional care because of stigma and general difficulty accessing mental health services.

However, emerging evidence indicates that the WHO's advocated strategy, task-shifting, is showing promising benefits in improving outcomes for mental health including self-harm thoughts and attempted suicide in low- and middle-income countries. Task-shifting involves the rational redistribution of tasks among health workforce teams. Specific tasks are moved, where appropriate, from highly qualified health workers to health workers with shorter training and fewer quali-fications in order to make more efficient use of the available human resources for healthcare (WHO, 2008, p. 2). Designed originally to expand and strengthen health workforce to increase access to HIV and AIDS care (particularly in low- and middle-income countries), task-shifting has been modelled recently to ex-pand cost-effective access to mental healthcare in similar settings. The services are offered through primary-level workers or non-specialist people who receive some mental health training, including primary healthcare professionals, commu-nity volunteers, nurses, physicians, lay health workers, and other community mem-bers, including teachers, traditional leaders, and social workers (van Ginneken et al., 2021). Primary-level workers deliver these intervention services alone or in collaboration with specialists for care of persons living with or experiencing mental problems or suicide-influencing distress. Ultimately, these primary-level workers or community health workers are tasked with delivering both optimal psychological and pharmacological treatments and other novel community-level interventions, across various setting—such as places of worship, homes, schools, community centres, and primary healthcare facilities.

In summary

- While therapy may be a response to self-harm, people value therapy that takes account of them as a person with whatever problems or feelings they have.
- A safety plan readily provides a list of actions that someone can take during a crisis associated with high risk of self-harm.
- Social skills, self-harm screening practices, and problem-solving skills training have been found to show potential in reducing self-harm among young people in detention.
- Enforcing non-discriminatory clauses in the healthcare system can promote equity and professional (mental) health-seeking among sexual and gender minority population.
- Task-shifting is showing promising benefits in improving mental health outcomes including self-harm thoughts and attempted suicide in low- and middle-income countries.

REFERENCES

Briggs, S., Netuveli, G., Gould, N., Gkaravella, A., Gluckman, N., Kangogyere, P., . . . Lindner, R. (2019). The effectiveness of psychoanalytic/psychodynamic psychotherapy for reducing suicide attempts and self-harm: systematic review and meta-analysis. *The British Journal of Psychiatry*, 214(6), 320–328. doi:10.1192/bjp.2019.33

Carter, A., Butler, A., Willoughby, M., Janca, E., Kinner, S. A., Southalan, L., Fazel, S., & Borschmann, R. (2022). Interventions to reduce suicidal thoughts and behaviours among people in contact with the criminal justice system: a global systematic review. *EClinicalMedicine*, *44*, 101266. https://doi.org/10.1016/j.eclinm.2021.101266

Cox, G., & Hetrick, S. (2017). Psychosocial interventions for self-harm, suicidal ideation and suicide attempt in children and young people: What? How? Who? and Where? *BMJ Mental Health*, *20*(2), 35–40. https://doi.org/10.1136/eb-2017-102667

Edelson, S. M., Johnson, J., & Rensselaer, A. V. (Eds.). (2016). *Understanding and treating self-injurious behavior in autism: a multi-disciplinary perspective*. London: Jessica Kingsley Publishers.

Jahoda, A., Hastings, R., Hatton, C., Cooper, S.-A., McMeekin, N., Dagnan, D., Appleton, K., Scott, K., Fulton, L., & Jones, R. (2018). Behavioural activation versus guided self-help for depression in adults with learning disabilities: the BeatIt RCT. *Health Technology Assessment*, *22*(53), 1–130. https://doi.org/10.3310/hta22530

Stefanopoulou, E., Hogarth, H., Taylor, M., Russell-Haines, K., Lewis, D., & Larkin, J. (2020). Are digital interventions effective in reducing suicidal ideation and self-harm? A systematic review. *Journal of Mental Health*, *29*(2), 207–216. https://doi.org/10.1080/09638237.2020.1714009

van Ginneken, N., Chin, W. Y., Lim, Y. C., Ussif, A., Singh, R., Shahmalak, U., Purgato, M., Rojas-García, A., Uphoff, E., & McMullen, S. (2021). Primary-level worker interventions for the care of people living with mental disorders and distress in low-and middle-income countries. *Cochrane Database of Systematic Reviews* (8). https://doi.org/10.1002/14651858.CD009149.pub3

WHO (2008). *Task shifting: rational redistribution of tasks among health workforce teams. Global recommendations and guidelines*. World Health Organization.

CHAPTER 5

Part 3
The person-centred approach to self-harm

Self-management approaches

KEY POINTS:
• Basic self-care includes attention to healthy diet, sleep, alcohol, and drug use.
• A crisis plan should include specific actions to alleviate stress and its effects.
• A longer-term plan can help articulate goals and develop effective ways to cope.
• Friends, family, and others may be a resource if actively involved.
• Online or written resources may be helpful if they are professionally prepared and used thoughtfully.

Not everybody who self-harms has access to professional help or wants to talk to somebody else. This is especially true for young people, who can be reluctant to confide in others. They may fear loss of privacy or that there will be some intrusive response that isn't what they want for themselves. As a result, self-management forms an important part of the response to self-harm. Indeed, most people are already trying, or have tried, to do something to resolve their problems. A useful starting place is therefore to review the range of self-management approaches available and those already tried, building on those found successful and adding new ones at a manageable rate.

Basic self-care

Most self-harm takes place against a background of low mood, which can be associated with problems of basic self-care including poor sleep habits, physical inactivity, overeating or irregular eating, and use of alcohol or drugs for their mood-altering properties. Such poor self-care can exacerbate low mood and low self-esteem and can impede problem-solving abilities. So, although it may not seem like the main problem it is worth supporting change if it is possible.

Sleep hygiene—poor sleep can increase vulnerability to self-harm, as those who are sleep deprived are more likely to be emotionally labile and impulsive (Hysing et al., 2015). Adequate sleep hygiene can help to reduce the risk of further self-harm and improve emotional regulation. Good sleep hygiene includes avoiding stimulants such as caffeine late in the day and near bedtime, or sedating substances including alcohol, that can impair REM sleep. Establishing and maintaining a regular sleep and wake schedule and limiting screen time before bedtime are important in developing a sleep routine. Other activities that can be incorporated into sleep hygiene include engaging in calming activities before bed, such as yoga or reading, and avoiding stressful activities before bedtime.

Healthy eating—while eating healthily is often associated with physical health it can also be helpful for those who self-harm. Eating healthily can help improve mental well-being, providing a sense of control. It can also help reinforce a sense of self-care and self-worth, which are often lacking in those who self-harm. Eating nutritious foods can also provide a source of energy which can help to reduce feelings of exhaustion and fatigue that can increase the risk of self-harm. Eating healthily means avoiding snacking, cheap high-calorie junk food or drinks. The individual should be encouraged to make the time to prepare a good meal, reducing reliance on store-bought unhealthy snacks.

Healthy eating can also be used to encourage positive social connections. For example, joining friends and family to eat can help a person to feel connected and supported, which can be beneficial for those who self-harm. It can also help to combat feelings of loneliness that can increase the risk of self-harm.

In order to make the most of healthy eating as a way of self-care, it is important to develop a healthy relationship with food. This involves understanding the importance of nutrition and balance, as well as developing self-aware eating habits. This means being aware of what you are eating and how it makes you feel, and being mindful of feelings of guilt or shame that can often accompany unhealthy eating.

Physical activity—keeping physically active and exercising can reduce stress and improve mood, with the effect being greatest for those engaging in moderate to vigorous intensity exercise for at least 30 minutes per day (Dunn et al., 2005; Pearce et al., 2022; Vancampfort et al., 2018). For a sustained routine, physical activity does not have to be heavy exercise; biking or (brisk) walking every day should yield desirable positive physical effects and improved mental state.

Physical activity can also provide a disruptive or competing activity when dealing with thoughts of self-harm as it requires focus and can act as an outlet for emotions.

Physical activity can provide a sense of control and mastery, and a sense of accomplishment and confidence as it may create a sense of self-efficacy. Additionally, it can provide a sense of community and social support—where one engages in exercise with other people—which can be beneficial for individuals who feel isolated and alone. In addition to the mental health benefits, physical activity has also been found to provide physical benefits such as improved physical strength and endurance, which can improve self-confidence and self-esteem. Physical activity may provide a healthy outlet for aggression and frustration, which can be beneficial for individuals who are struggling with anger or other intense emotions.

CHAPTER 6

Drugs and alcohol—both drug and alcohol use and self-harm are described by some people as coping strategies. Many individuals struggling with self-harm turn to drugs and alcohol as a form of self-care. They may believe that using drugs and alcohol will provide them with the relief they need to cope with their distress. However, using drugs and alcohol as a form of self-care can be less helpful and is not an effective way to manage difficult emotions. For some the drinking of alcohol in itself is a kind of indirect self-harm. Both alcohol and drug use can change emotional states, lower inhibitions, and can contribute to sudden dips in mood, thereby increasing the risk for self-harm. Excessive use can lead to dependence, which can damage physical health and worsen mental health problems, strain social relationships and lead to financial hardship.

Physical care—minor self-injuries, such as cuts, scratches, or bruises, may be treated at home with simple first aid supplies like cleaning wipes, cold pack, or bandages. Seeking medical treatment should not be avoided if needed—where injuries are severe and threaten bodily function, for example, through damage to nerves or tendons, or where scarring is likely.

It is important not to share objects or items used for self-injury, so that the risk of infection, for example with hepatitis or HIV, can be reduced. If the individual does not wish to stop self-injury then it can be important to offer advice about what has been called *harm-minimization*, which typically involves awareness of basic anatomy to avoid damage to important structures and understanding good wound care to avoid infection or avoidable scarring.

Physical care may involve paying attention to existing scars. A few people do not mind exposing scars, for example by wearing short-sleeved tops, but most wish to hide them if only to avoid intrusive staring or questions from others. Apart from clothing, make-up may be helpful and there are sites online to advise about camouflage make-up. For those who can afford it, camouflage tattooing or surgical scar removal may be an option.

Emotional self-care—basic self-care need not involve just stopping things. Treats are good—music, saving for clothes, visit a favourite place, watch a film, or whatever. The idea is to do something that can help boost self-esteem by conveying a personal message about being worth the effort.

Crisis planning

Experiencing an emotional crisis means being exposed to what feels like overwhelming thoughts and feelings—typically in a situation that calls for some immediate response. While there is no right or wrong way to feel or think when in a crisis, how one responds during a crisis or what steps one takes in response to the crisis are important. The idea here is to make a crisis response plan. This can be easier with another person but can be undertaken alone if another person is not available or trusted to help.

CHAPTER 6

Crisis planning is a proactive approach to managing immediate stressors, the emotional distress they generate and the resultant risk of further self-harm. The crisis plan outlines actions to be used if and when a person begins to experience intense negative emotions that could lead to self-harm. By creating a plan ahead of time, individuals can feel empowered to take steps to manage their distress and prevent self-harm. This can be especially beneficial for those who have difficulty recognizing their own emotions or lack the skills to manage them effectively. Crisis planning can also help individuals build self-confidence and self-efficacy, by providing them with tangible steps to take in moments of distress. Ultimately, crisis planning can also be a form of self-care. Below are five ideas that can be included in a (written) crisis plan:

1. **Allow watchful waiting**—put differently, stop and think it through; do not act at once or impulsively. Doing things in a panic can make matters worse. When the dust has settled it is easier to think about what actually needs doing. The idea of allowing watchful waiting can contribute to buying time, during which self-harm thoughts or urges might subside but also allows for thinking about helpful next steps by defining the problems and identifying the key problem to work on; identifying some different possible solutions to the identified problem and thinking about which one of the identified possible solutions looks like a place to start. This preliminary thinking, undertaken in the 'time-out' created by watchful waiting, can usefully feed into more structured approaches to problem-solving that are outlined in Chapter 7.

2. **Seek company and support**—it is important to remember it is fine to ask for help by making connection with trusted others. Examples include getting in touch with a trusted friend or family member, contacting a support group, or contacting a mental healthcare provider. Other resources may include crisis (call or text) lines offering help. It may be also helpful to write a list of all the people, organizations, and websites that the individual could go to for help when finding things difficult.

A worry that many people have is about how any disclosure about self-harm will be received. Planning disclosure includes recognizing that it does not need to involve confiding too much about the nature of or reasons for current problems. The important message is to be in control of what is said, which might mean speaking only about stresses leading to the current crisis, or only sharing something about current distress—confiding about self-harm can come later if desired.

3. **Consider disrupting or substitution of actions**—the idea here is to interrupt the urge to self-harm by engaging in something else. Numerous strategies are available: call a friend for a chat; do something physical—run, dance, jump rope, hit a punching bag, play with a pet; walk in nature; make noise (shout, play an instrument, bang on pots and pans); write a

letter about how you are feeling, then destroy it; massage your hands; take a bath or hot shower; tidy up; weed the garden.

An alternative is use of diversionary strategies—performing an action that is similar to self-harm and may be painful but does not result in injury. Some diversionary strategies have been suggested: drawing on the body instead of cutting; flicking elastic or rubber bands on the inside of the wrists; holding or squeezing ice cubes or having a very cold shower; eating something with a strong taste such as chilli. Many people do not like to use disruptive or diversionary techniques. They can feel trivializing ('just take your mind off it for a bit and it will go away') or do not work as plausible or effective substitutes. For those who do want to try them, they can be thought of as ways of building in time so that alternatives to damaging self-harm can be contemplated.

4. ***Plan ahead for predictable provocations***—there is often a pattern to crises in personal life such as family arguments, abuse from peers, harassment—stresses that arise from long-standing difficulties in relationships or personal circumstances. Planning ahead is therefore rather like problem-solving; that is, thinking ahead about what crisis is likely to happen in the future, defining what exactly the issue is and thinking about potential solutions.

5. ***Develop a safety plan***—A safety plan is a document that helps and guides someone when they are experiencing thoughts of self-harm, to support them to avoid a state of intense self-harm crisis. Anyone in a trusting relationship with the person at risk of self-harm can help make the safety plan, they do not need to be a professional. A safety plan is made (preferably written) when a person is not experiencing intense thoughts of self-harm. It may be written after a self-harm crisis, but not during, as at this time a person may be unable to think clearly. Details of a safety plan are discussed in Chapter 5 of this volume. Copies of the safety plan should be easily accessible; it can be paper-based or stored on a phone. Essentially, a safety plan is a list of coping strategies and sources of support that a person can use before or during a self-harm crisis.

   It includes:
   • Coping strategies
   • Personal warning signs
   • Ways to stay safe at the workplace or school
   • People or places that can provide a distraction
   • Trusted persons they can contact for help, and
   • Ways to keep the environment safe (including removing or limiting access to dangerous objects and substances).

CHAPTER 6

So far, we have discussed the self-management in the short-term: dealing with the stresses leading to episodes of self-harm and the act of self-harm itself. However, self-management can also involve taking a longer view and we discuss that in the next part of this chapter.

Articulate longer-term goals and plans

Taking stock

Considering personal goals and values

This does not mean indulging in fantasy, but reviewing what might be practically possible given the circumstances. People often don't articulate these thoughts for fear of being dismissed or of setting themselves up for failure. Examples might include returning to education that was interrupted by personal problems or left early, changing employment, or moving to live in a new venue. The initial stage of taking stock does not involve achieving these goals—simply acknowledging that they form a part of personal ambitions for the future.

Identifying key people

Family and peer group may be resources; consider the barriers to using them as such. They may also be the source of stress. How can that be resolved? Sometimes by taking action (interpersonal problem-solving) but sometimes the only solution is distancing from damaging relationships.

Reviewing barriers to change

People often feel stuck or hopeless about changing. They may feel there are practical barriers such as lack of money or work skills, or the problem may be more motivational—a sense that any attempt to change will inevitably fail so isn't worth the effort. Taking stock includes analysing these barriers and questioning what they are exactly as opposed to what they are assumed to be. Is it really true that 'nobody wants to help me' or that 'I am unemployable'? How important is money to achievement of a particular goal and how much money is needed to make it possible to make a start?

An alternative approach is to concentrate not on barriers, which can feel rather demoralizing, but on what works rather than what doesn't. Asking this question, sometimes called affirmative inquiry, can lead to different ways of thinking about the problems to be tackled (why did this work when that didn't?) or the solutions to be tried.

Future planning

It is worth considering three resources that somebody might use in their self-management—optimizing their practical social support; approaching third-sector (voluntary) organizations; using online resources.

CHAPTER 6

Family, friends, and peer support

The ability to marshal social support depends upon three conditions. One of course is the availability of people who are prepared to form part of the individual's social network. The other two depend upon the individual and involve developing trust in others. In typical circumstances trust in others (a central feature of what has been called social capital) is built on ties of mutual obligation or kinship ties. If these are lacking, then trust has to be developed through experience.

One consequence of participation in a trusting social network is the opportunity it allows for confiding—willingness to take the risk of sharing sensitive or personal thoughts with another. Confiding relationships have been shown to be emotionally protective in the presence of stressful events.

The other major type of support is practical (sometimes called instrumental) support. It takes many forms and can include financial support, help with transport or housing, or more intangible acts like providing information and advice.

As indicated earlier in this section, young people in particular can be reluctant, even with encouragement, to confide in others. They may fear loss of privacy or that there will be some intrusive response that is not what they want for themselves. However, family, friends, and others may be a resource if actively involved. Confiding in others can be helpful in managing and reducing the risk of self-harm. By opening up to a trusted person about the challenges they are facing, individuals can gain the support and understanding they need in order to cope with the issues that lead or have led to self-harm. Confiding in others can also help to reduce feelings of shame and guilt, which are often associated with self-harm. Furthermore, it can provide individuals with a sense of connection and belonging, which is crucial in managing the psychological and emotional distress that can lead to self-harm.

The power of peer support in tackling the issue of self-harm should not be underestimated. Connecting with peers who understand and can relate to the challenges someone is facing can provide invaluable support and comfort. Peer support can also provide individuals with a safe space to talk openly and honestly about their experiences, enabling them to identify and address the underlying causes of their self-harm. Peer support can help to reduce stigma and create a sense of community and solidarity, allowing individuals to feel less alone in their struggle.

Third-sector (voluntary, non-statutory) organizations

Third-sector (voluntary) organizations are usually organized with the aim of helping a particular vulnerable group in society. They do not necessarily focus on mental health or self-harm, but because self-harm so often has causes in the social world, they may be offering help. Examples will vary locally and can include:

Age-related: may help lonely elderly, the young, and vulnerable
Physical health and disability
Mental health

Addictions
Social welfare—debt, housing
Education and training, skills
Religious practice and support

There may be barriers or problems associated with accessing third-sector groups. For example, religious groups can offer support but you may have to subscribe to certain beliefs or ways of behaving. Many organizations are reluctant to become involved with somebody for whom substance misuse is an active issue. People without experience of it can find self-harm alarming and assume that it is a sign of problems that are too great for them to help. It is worth exploring some of these questions with the individual and (perhaps) with the organization rather than making a referral simply in the hope that it will work. As with all interventions, the individual should approach with an open mind—trying something to see if it helps allows for the possibility that if it doesn't work out, then it need not then lead to a sense of personal failure or being let down.

Online resources and social media

Research into the mental health benefits and risks of internet use is still emerging. Much public discussion has centred on the idea that exposure to certain online content related to self-harm can heighten the risk of self-harm by encouraging imitation, triggering urges, normalizing self-harm, and inducing a sense of competition. However, the online world and digital media can also be a potentially valuable resource for persons who need help when experiencing self-harm urges or crisis, as online media platforms and social media sites are readily and easily accessible and are mostly used by young people. Social media content in particular has been shown to have both harmful and helpful effects for persons experiencing self-harm. In the following subsections, we draw on the key findings of a published systematic review of the evidence from recent studies (Brennan et al., 2022).

Some mechanisms of harm from social media

For most content it is not always possible to attribute harm arising from the content itself but it may be harmful to some depending on the context in which it is accessed. However, some mechanisms of harm are easy to understand and recognize. They are recognizable in the overt or explicit harmful content of posts:

- Explicit verbal encouragement to act or to escalate severity of actions (including that found in 'games' or challenges);
- Online self-harm or suicide pacts;
- Circulation of manifestly disturbing content (such as live streams);
- Offering detail of methods;
- Trolling or abusing posters who are expressing personal distress.

CHAPTER 6

Less clearcut is content where the effect may be less well established or may depend very much on context, an ambiguity that arises because posts do not contain the explicit messages outlined above but may carry similar implicit messages.

- The likelihood of imitative or copycat behaviour, sometimes called spreading by contagion;
- The role of posts (texts or images) about self-harm in normalizing or glamorizing—that is, presenting self-harm as a natural or desirable, even chic, response to circumstances;
- The role of images in reawakening impulses to self-harm, sometimes referred to as triggering with the assumption that such impulses are already there but somehow suppressed or inhibited until a new image is presented.

More indirectly, social media posts about self-harm and related emotional problems may induce a lowering of mood, especially when exposure is prolonged and repeated, immersing the viewer to the exclusion other social cues.

Some mechanisms of benefit from social media

Responses from those who self-harm can tell us of a number of benefits from accessing self-harm content on social media:

- Using forums to talk as a means of clarifying and sharing a personal story in a non-judgemental environment provides a sense of relief and reduces stigma.
- Exploring and defining an identity.
- Seeking and offering practical advice; online access to good-quality advice and support is important given that self-harm and suicidal thinking are often difficult to talk about directly.
- Vicarious experience online may reduce direct personal urges to harm.
- Receiving emotional support and recovery messages from people who have (or at least are perceived to have) the same experiences.

Seeking and using professional help

Knowing how to access and use professional help is part of self-management. Seeking professional help may include seeing a counsellor, therapist, psychologist, or psychiatrist, or joining a support group. These professionals can provide individualized treatment to help address the underlying issues causing the self-harm, such as depression or anxiety. For example, a therapist may use cognitive-behavioural therapy to help change thought patterns and behaviours that can lead to self-harm. It is also important to use professional help to create a plan to reduce or stop self-harm. As discussed earlier (and mainly in Chapter 5 of

CHAPTER 6

this volume) this plan should, among other important things, focus on developing healthier coping strategies, identifying triggers that can lead to self-harm and what specific steps or actions one can take when the triggers occur.

However, people sometimes avoid seeking professional help for fear of loss of confidentiality, involvement of people (like parents) they do not want involved. Also, people may be doubtful about the usefulness and helpfulness of what is on offer; there are lots of myths about mental health services. In certain instances, though, seeking professional care becomes inevitable—for example, where the severity and physical consequences of self-poisoning or self-injury is dangerous. Once committed to it is important to follow the treatment plan and stick with therapy appointments, practice and use coping skills learned in therapy, and adhere to medication as directed.

In low- and middle-income countries what is on offer in terms of mental healthcare towards self-harm intervention and prevention may vary considerably, mainly due to the shortage or unavailability of trained specialists and professionals. As outlined earlier (in Chapter 5 of this volume), what is emerging is that in low- and middle-income countries primary-level workers deliver mental health (intervention) services alone or in collaboration with specialists across various settings such as places of worship, homes, schools, community centres, and primary healthcare facilities.

In summary

- Not everybody who self-harms has access to professional help or wants to talk to somebody else, but knowing how to access and use professional help is part of self-management.
- Good sleep hygiene can help to reduce the risk of further self-harm and improve emotional regulation.
- Physical activity can provide a disruptive or competing activity when dealing with thoughts of self-harm.
- Both alcohol and drugs can change emotional states, lower inhibitions, and can contribute to sudden dips in mood, thereby increasing the risk for self-harm.
- By creating a plan ahead of time, individuals can feel empowered to take steps to manage their distress and prevent self-harm.
- Besides dealing with immediate stresses leading to episodes of self-harm, self-management can also involve taking a longer view.

CHAPTER 6

REFERENCES

Brennan, C., Saraiva, S., Mitchell, E., Melia, R., Campbell, L., King, N., & House, A. (2022). Self-harm and suicidal content online, harmful or helpful? A systematic review of the recent evidence. *Journal of Public Mental Health, 21*(1), 57–69. https://doi.org/10.1108/JPMH-09-2021-0118

Dunn, A. L., Trivedi, M. H., Kampert, J. B., Clark, C. G., & Chambliss, H. O. (2005). Exercise treatment for depression: efficacy and dose response. *American Journal of Preventive Medicine, 28*(1), 1–8. https://doi.org/10.1016/j.amepre.2004.09.003

Hysing, M., Sivertsen, B., Stormark, K. M., & O'Connor, R. C. (2015). Sleep problems and self-harm in adolescence. *The British Journal of Psychiatry, 207*(4), 306–312. https://doi.org/10.1192/bjp.bp.114.146514

Pearce, M., Garcia, L., Abbas, A., Strain, T., Schuch, F. B., Golubic, R., Kelly, P., Khan, S., Utukuri, M., & Laird, Y. (2022). Association between physical activity and risk of depression: a systematic review and meta-analysis. *JAMA Psychiatry, 79*(6), 550–559. https://doi.org/10.1001/jamapsychiatry.2022.0609

Vancampfort, D., Hallgren, M., Firth, J., Rosenbaum, S., Schuch, F. B., Mugisha, J., Probst, M., Van Damme, T., Carvalho, A. F., & Stubbs, B. (2018). Physical activity and suicidal ideation: a systematic review and meta-analysis. *Journal of Affective Disorders, 225*, 438–448. https://doi.org/10.1016/j.jad.2017.08.070

The personal encounter with self-harm

> **KEY POINTS**
>
> - An immediate response is to review
>   - The need for treatment of physical consequences of poisoning or injury
>   - Current mental state assessment focused on symptoms, suicidal thinking, and safety
>   - The current social circumstances and who knows.
> - Further assessment will cover wider social circumstances, psychological factors, and consequences of self-harm.
> - Care planning includes both an immediate response and a longer-term plan that includes mobilizing all available resources.
> - A person-centred approach includes sensitive use of language, a non-judgemental style, cultural sensitivity, and confidence in discussing all aspects of self-harm.

Up to this stage we have been reviewing what is known about self-harm in general terms. In this chapter we discuss practical aspects of the response to an individual who has confided that they have self-harmed or self-harm has been identified in some other way.

The immediate response

First things first. At an initial contact it is always important to start with a few personal basics: do not judge the person for harming themselves; be sensitive to personal, social and cultural circumstances, try to from a collaborative and therapeutic alliance; discuss confidentiality.

The immediate task is then to make an assessment of the individual's physical, psychological, and social safety and well-being. Exactly what form this takes will depend upon how recent the last episode was and what form it took.

Physical assessment

It may be that the most pressing need is to assess physical health—if for example somebody has recently taken an overdose of medication or has done something to injure themselves, then the outcome may depend upon prompt treatment.

After self-injury the problems that need a response are non-healing, bleeding, or infected wounds. Even if they are not that recent, the risks from uncontrolled infection or from scarring can be severe. A quick visual inspection is usually enough to allow a decision about whether medical help should be sought.

In relation to self-poisoning, it is desirable that anybody who has taken an overdose in the last 24-48 hours has a medical assessment. That is because there are some drugs for which there are time deadlines for providing treatment before damage is done, even if the person who has taken the tablets has no symptoms when seen; a common one is paracetamol. Medical assessment is also desirable when an overdose is said to have been taken longer ago, if symptoms are present. Common early symptoms of poisoning are given in Table 7.1.

Mental state assessment

Mental state may change quite rapidly at around the time of an episode of self-harm. A full assessment may not be possible because the individual is unwell or if the circumstances do not allow easily for a discussion about sensitive matters. However, if at all possible it is worth trying to establish early on if there are aspects of the current mental state that suggest an immediate risk. These fall into three main categories:

- Symptoms of severe mental illness—especially psychotic symptoms like hearing voices or delusions. They are uncommon but important to identify;
- Strongly negative thoughts especially about the self, such as hopelessness or a sense of personal worthlessness;
- Continuing thoughts about suicide, especially thinking about how to act on suicidal thoughts or plans to do so, *even if a previous act of self-harm is not described as suicidal.*

Social assessment

A person seen after an act of self-harm, or who is thinking about self-harm, should never be thought of in isolation. Most of the help that people need for self-harm will come not from professional services but from informal sources (Iyengar et al., 2018). An early review of somebody's personal circumstances will be aimed at identifying:

- Who is involved in their immediate social network—family, friends, significant others? That is, who do they live with or see regularly?
- Who knows about the self-harm and in what detail?
- Who does the individual think of as a potential helper, even if they haven't yet confided in them? And who can be contacted now, as part of an immediate action plan?

Table 7.1 Common early symptoms of poisoning

Drug	Symptoms and signs
Paracetamol	**Note: people who have ingested paracetamol are frequently asymptomatic. People who are suspected of taking a paracetamol overdose should be urgently admitted to hospital.** Nausea and vomiting usually settle within 24 hours. If these continue, often with the development of right abdominal pain and tenderness, this suggests the development of liver damage. People may also present with coma, a reduced level of consciousness, or respiratory depression, if they have taken paracetamol with a drug that reduces the level of consciousness, such as opioids (for example, a combined paracetamol/opioid preparation) or alcohol.
Aspirin	Hyperventilation, tinnitus, deafness, flushing, and sweating.
Tricyclic and related antidepressants	Dry mouth, seizures, drowsiness, cardiac rhythm problems.
Selective serotonin re-uptake inhibitors (SSRIs)	Nausea, vomiting, agitation, tremor, drowsiness, tachycardia. There may be convulsions.
Beta-blockers	Slow heart, fainting, heart rhythm problems. Other features may include drowsiness, confusion, convulsions.
Iron salts	Nausea, vomiting, diarrhoea, abdominal pain, vomiting, and rectal bleeding.
Benzodiazepines	Drowsiness, unsteadiness, and slurred speech.
Antimalarials (quinine, chloroquine, hydroxychloroquine)	Rapid onset of life-threatening heart rhythm problems and seizures. Note: overdose with these is extremely dangerous and difficult to treat. The person should be referred to hospital urgently.
Antipsychotic drugs	Sinus tachycardia, arrhythmias, hypothermia, hypotension, reduced consciousness, and respiratory depression. Dystonic reactions may be seen with therapeutic doses. Seizures in severe cases.
Amphetamines	Initially excessive activity, wakefulness, hallucinations, paranoia, and hypertension. Later there may be convulsions, hyperthermia, exhaustion, and coma.
Cocaine	Agitation, hypertension, tachycardia, dilated pupils, hallucinations, hyperthermia, hypertonia, and hyperreflexia and cardiac effects such as chest pain, arrhythmias, myocardial infarction.
Opioids, e.g. morphine, heroin	Drowsiness, coma, respiratory depression, pinpoint pupils.
Methylenedioxymethamphetamine (MDMA, ecstasy)	Delirium, coma, hyperthermia, rhabdomyolysis, acute renal failure, acute hepatitis, disseminated intravascular coagulation, adult respiratory distress syndrome, hyperreflexia, hypotension, and intracerebral haemorrhage; hyponatraemia, convulsions, ventricular arrhythmias, delirium, coma.

The purpose of this initial assessment is to decide first who needs immediate professional attention for the physical effects of self-harm, or for symptoms that might amount to mental disorder. If immediate professional referral is not indicated, then help will likely come so-called informal sources, which should be identified so that the individual can be encouraged or supported in mobilizing them.

The next step: a more detailed assessment

Once the immediate safety of the individual has been established, it is possible to make a more comprehensive assessment and develop a plan.

Social assessment

Most episodes of self-harm are a response to recent circumstances (events or crises) and when asked, most people can give a reasonably clear account of the events leading up to the self-harm. Using a checklist may be helpful in encouraging a discussion of these problems and in indicating how common such problems are. There is an example in Chapter 3. There are certain types of stressors that are sufficiently common and severe that they should be asked about specifically even if they are not volunteered:

> *Physical or sexual abuse victimization*, including a question about the relation to the perpetrator. This is especially important if the perpetrator is a family member or close other, or has access to other vulnerable people—for example, if they are a teacher or care worker;
> *Coercive control*, where the victim is denied independence, for example, financially or socially;
> *Emotional or physical neglect* from somebody who should be in a caring role.

There is almost always more to the story than can be understood by a description of recent events. In the background are likely to be past events or more long-standing difficulties; they are important because they often provide the context out of which recent events have developed and they can give those recent events their meaning.

It may be that the individual does not describe any recent events to which self-harm was a response. In this situation, the response to the question 'why self-harm now' is likely to be a description of personal feelings—because somebody feels worthless or hopeless or deserving of punishment. The origin of these feelings will be in earlier experiences and so an exploration of the personal and social background is still relevant.

Recent and more distant events and difficulties typically, although not always, involve other people either as the source of problems or as a resource in dealing with those problems (Fliege et al., 2009). So a part of social assessment is biographical. Both now and at important times in the person's past life, what are the key relationships with kin, friends, and peers. What is the nature of their relationship with the key people they mention? Is it friendly and helpful? Or are they a source of stress in the individual's life?

In exploring the answers to these questions, two key ideas are useful to keep in mind. One is about the nature of *support* and the other is about the nature of closeness and *confiding*.

Broadly, support can be thought of as practical or emotional. Practical support might involve, for example, helping with somewhere to sleep, or providing food, clothing or money. It might involve giving information or advice or introducing somebody to a helping agency. Emotional support is more intangible. It can involve treating somebody with respect, being available to listen when they want to talk, or simply spending time with somebody who is lonely or frightened. A balance of the two approaches is usually best.

Confiding involves talking freely to somebody. Sometimes it is a one-off episode, not repeated if the response is unhelpful or actively rejecting in some way. On the other hand, it can become a defining part of a close relationship with somebody else who is trusted to offer understanding and non-judgemental emotional support, or perhaps to respond with practical support. A completely confiding relationship involves being able to share everything with another person, however apparently embarrassing or shameful it might feel to do so. In fact completely confiding relationships are quite rare. For example, in a study in the UK, most people named only one or two people in whom they confided completely. Men are less likely to confide freely than women.

Social support comes most frequently from other people—friends, family, professional contacts like teachers or social workers. Emotional support and confiding are most likely to come from somebody whom the individual trusts, while practical support including information can come from a wider range of sources. For many younger people the internet is a source of information and advice, not always good of course, like all information and advice. Even emotional support may be obtained via social media although it is likely to be more superficial and unreliable than emotional support from a trusted and caring friend or family member.

Social support and confiding relationships are both protective against depression and it is therefore important to consider, when asking about relationships, which of them have either of these characteristics.

Mental state assessment

If somebody confides about self-harm it is important to gain a picture of their mental state, both at the time and in the past. However, an overdetailed or elaborate examination can be off-putting to somebody who might want to talk about what is happening in their life, so some care is needed in keeping questions to an acceptable number and range. The main features to cover are (see Table 7.2):

Table 7.2 Mental state assessment

	Example	Importance
Appearance and behaviour	Evidence of levels of self-care; oddities of dress or gesture	Can give clues to neglect by self or others, or to otherwise hidden mental illness
Speech	Speed and spontaneity	May indicate social awkwardness or lack of trust, or an underlying disturbance of thinking
Mood	Especially depression, anxiety, or irritability and anger	People often hide how low in mood they are, unless asked directly
Thought	Especially negative thoughts about self (such as worthlessness, guilt) the present (such as loneliness) and the future (hopelessness, helplessness)	Can indicate risk for future episodes of self-harm and for suicide
Cognition (form and content)	Confusion, poor memory	In older people can indicate onset of dementia, in younger people often the effects of drugs or alcohol
Judgement	Accurate assessment of current situation	Poor judgement can impair problem-solving or indicate more severe mental illness

People who self-harm often have had previous mental health problems. The commonest are episodes of depression and problems cause by misuse of alcohol and drugs. They also often have previous episodes of self-harm. More useful than just asking about events and their dates is asking about the circumstances under which previous mental health problems and previous episodes of self-harm occurred. The individual's account can help to shed light on their current problems and the way they respond to them.

Assessment of coping and help-seeking

Hardly anybody is completely passive in response to stressful experiences and challenges. What has the individual been doing to try and cope with current circumstances, using their individual and social resources?

What has the individual done themselves practically to solve any recent problems? Have they, for example, sought information that will help them? Or taken steps to sort out housing problems, or contacted the police if they are being threatened? How have they, using their own resources, tried to manage their emotional state? What do they do when they feel low in mood or anxious and there is nobody around to turn to?

In relation to social resources, who have they turned to for help, either practical or emotional? Different people can serve different functions in somebody's life. You might accept a lift from somebody or borrow money from them when you would not rely on them for emotional support.

Previous crises and how the individual responded can be a useful guide. When things have gone wrong before what has the individual done? Is there a pattern to how they deal with events?

- Active coping or a tendency to avoid issues and 'wait and see', hoping troubles pass;
- Reliance on self and personal resources or seeking help from others;
- Taking a practical problem-solving approach, or using mainly emotional coping?

These questions may reveal a certain 'style' of responding to stressful circumstances. If it has worked in the past, then the question is—why not now? If it has not worked well, is the individual recycling ineffective strategies when they could be trying new ones?

Formulation (explaining the self-harm episode)

Rarely can self-harm be viewed as simply a symptom of mental illness, a response to delusions for example. The more useful way to think of it is as a response to personal and social adversity. It may be a sign that other ways of coping have not been entirely successful, or it may in fact be a part of somebody's coping repertoire. This idea, that self-harm can be seen as having a purpose for the individual, is relatively new and it is extremely important in understanding the individual and how to help them.

How can self-harm be seen as a meaningful response to circumstances? We outlined possible answers to this question in Chapter 3. The issue may be explored with open questions first, for example:

> Given all that has happened to you and how you felt, can you explain why you self-harmed? Can you say what you were thinking about self-harm just before you did it? That is, what you thought about why you might self-harm, given everything that was going on?

By this stage in the assessment, some possibilities will be pretty clear and it can be worth following up by putting more specific possibilities to the individual:

> In this situation, people sometimes think of self-harm as a way of, for example, punishing themselves, or expressing angry feelings, or showing somebody else how you feel. Does that sound like it might apply to you?

CHAPTER 7

> **Box 7.1** ABC aid-memoire
>
> **Antecedents—what** was happening before the episode of self-harm?
>
> - Long-standing personal or social problems
> - Recent stressful events or difficulties
> - Personal mental state, thoughts, and feelings
>
> **Behaviour—what** did the individual do in the circumstances described?
>
> - Personal coping actions—practical and emotional
> - Use of external resources—people and impersonal
>
> **Consequences—what** has happened since the self-harm
>
> - Change in stressors
> - Change in other people
> - Change in the individual

Finally: taking stock

How have circumstances changed since the self-harm—either in the way the individual feels, or the behaviour of others, or the worsening or improvement of other stressors? Change might be, at least in part, a consequence of the self-harm or it might have depended upon entirely other factors.

In summary, one way to think of this assessment is using the example in Box 7.1.

Developing a plan

A plan needs to start with a clear statement of the aims of any actions. That means, what does the person hope to achieve? That might include:

- resolution of interpersonal problems (arguments, abuse, harassment)
- practical assistance with problems of living (housing, debt, legal problems)
- help with emotional difficulties (anxiety, depression)
- help with associated mental health problems (addictions, eating disorder)
- help with reducing or preventing self-harm

The means of achieving these aims are described elsewhere—in Chapters 5 and 6. The personal plan brings together the various elements outlined in an individual plan which should be:

- an immediate (crisis) plan
- a personal safety plan
- a self-management plan
- support with problem-solving strategies
- arrangements for more formal therapy

Unless the individual actively refuses it, some form of further contact is desirable to offer support with the plan and to check on well-being. A decision needs to be made about where that will be—at home or in some other domestic setting; in a school, community centre or other safe place; in a primary or secondary care clinical setting.

The personal interaction

Discussions about self-harm can be difficult for both parties. They can raise sensitive topics and worry about safety, as well as strong feelings. Care is needed in how they are conducted.

The key idea is to remain *person-centred in discussion and planning*. What do people value in discussions about self-harm?

- The *opportunity to share*—listening is therefore important, with questions and comments designed to encourage somebody who is reticent.
- The *physical space to talk and reflect*—involves finding a place that feels safe and private, and time to talk without feeling flustered or a nuisance.
- Maintaining *respectful boundaries*—people want a concerned but not over-intimate response, which can feel overwhelming rather than supportive.
- A *non-judgemental response*—people who self-harm are often fearful of the response they might get if others find out, or critical of the response they have had from others when they have confided. *Sensitive use of language* is therefore important, avoiding words that imply the individual is blameworthy, or weak or doing something wrong.
- *Genuine concern*—one of the common comments made by those who have not found the response to their self-harm helpful is that the response they received reflected the needs of the person they were with, rather than their own needs. For example, a professional might have seemed more interested in following procedures or filling out forms, or an informal confidant wanted to manage their own anxiety. Genuine concern involves a desire to understand and respond to the needs of the person who has self-harmed, as the primary aim of any interaction.
- *Confidence*—in talking about and dealing with self-harm can be difficult to communicate if the experience is new, but it should always be possible to convey the idea that the situation is manageable.
- *Cultural sensitivity*—includes an understanding of local and national influences on what might happen. For example, religious attitudes to suicide and attempted suicide may encourage thinking that it is shameful and something to be hidden, in countries where suicide is illegal fear of police involvement may be an issue. Where sexual minorities are poorly tolerated then gay or trans people may be especially wary of confiding.

Interestingly, these desired features of help are closely related to what have been called the non-specific or generic features of successful psychotherapies—active listening, non-judgemental understanding, and accepting attitude, follow-up, and continuity of care. An empathic and compassionate model of self-harm care, in which the concerns and needs of patients are valued and respected, along with continuity of care remain at the core of professional care for patients presenting with self-harm (Lindgren et al., 2018; Mughal et al., 2020; Mughal & Quinlivan, 2021).

In summary

- Self-harm can be viewed a symptom of mental illness, but a more useful way to think of it is as a response to personal and social adversity.
- A person seen after an act of self-harm, or who is thinking about self-harm, should never be thought of in isolation.
- One way to think of self-harm assessment is using an ABC *aide-memoire*: Antecedents, Behaviour, and Consequences.
- Providing a balance of practical and emotional support is usually best.
- At the core of professional care for patients presenting with self-harm is an empathic and compassionate model of continuity of care that values and respects patients' needs.

REFERENCES

Fliege, H., Lee, J.-R., Grimm, A., & Klapp, B. F. (2009). Risk factors and correlates of deliberate self-harm behavior: a systematic review. *Journal of Psychosomatic Research*, 66(6), 477–493. https://doi.org/10.1016/j.jpsychores.2008.10.013

Iyengar, U., Snowden, N., Asarnow, J. R., Moran, P., Tranah, T., & Ougrin, D. (2018). A further look at therapeutic interventions for suicide attempts and self-harm in adolescents: an updated systematic review of randomized controlled trials. *Frontiers in Psychiatry*, 9, 583. https://doi.org/10.3389/fpsyt.2018.00583

Lindgren, B.-M., Svedin, C. G., & Werkö, S. (2018). A systematic literature review of experiences of professional care and support among people who self-harm. *Archives of Suicide Research*, 22(2), 173–192. https://doi.org/10.1080/13811118.2017.1319309

Mughal, F., & Quinlivan, L. (2021). The need for compassionate self-harm services. *British Medical Journal*, 373, n1478. https://doi.org/10.1136/bmj.n1478

Mughal, F., Troya, M. I., Dikomitis, L., Chew-Graham, C. A., & Babatunde, O. O. (2020). Role of the GP in the management of patients with self-harm behaviour: a systematic review. *British Journal of General Practice*, 70(694), e364–e373. https://doi.org/10.3399/bjgp20X708257

CHAPTER 7

Looking to the future

KEY POINTS

- Self-harm rates continue to grow: it is estimated that up to one in five of young people have a personal history of self-harm by the time they reach 20 years old.
- Self-harm is now discussed as a public health problem in mainstream and academic media and also in social media.
- There is a need to look for social or cultural explanations, given the absence of a plausible physical explanation for self-harm at a population level.
- More specific culturally sensitive explanatory models of self-harm are needed to inform the formulation of preventive measures.
- Increasing the access to peer-support or online resources can contribute to addressing the mismatch between the large numbers of people who self-harm, and the much smaller number of professionals able to provide evidence-based interventions.

Despite more than half a century of observing self-harm in society there are several aspects of the phenomenon about which we have relatively little knowledge.

Self-harm as a social phenomenon

It was only in the years after World War 2 that self-harm emerged as an important public health (as opposed to individual) problem, initially recognized in the UK and North America. Rates increased dramatically in countries where data were being collected, such as the UK, where the recently nationalized health service made collection of statistics easier, at least for hospital attendances. Rates have continued to grow in the decades since, so that now it is estimated that up to one in five of young people have a history of self-harm by the time they reach age 20 (Rodway et al., 2016). Accurate figures from low- and middle-income countries have only more recently been collected, and where they have become available they paint a similar picture (Aggarwal et al., 2017; Quarshie et al., 2020).

It appears that what has happened is that self-harm has become endemic. That is, it is present consistently across time and across many countries. It is discussed as a public health problem in mainstream and academic media and it is a source of widespread comment and information sharing online and especially in social media. Physical causes are often sought to explain both epidemics and disorders that become endemic such as influenza (viral infection), lung cancer (cigarette smoking) or type 2 diabetes (diet and obesity). In the absence of a plausible physical explanation for self-harm at a population level, we must look for social and cultural explanations.

With this possibility in mind, it can reasonably be suggested that self-harm has become a socially and culturally recognized way of responding to stressful experiences and personal distress, and not simply a symptom of mental illness. Over the era during which self-harm has emerged there has been significant social changes in many countries—in family structure, urbanization, patterns of work, and living arrangements, and so on. It is difficult not to see all these things as related, and many of the explanations that individuals offer for self-harm can be linked to them—family and relationship problems, educational and employment challenges, and so on. Self-harm can then be seen as a response to the social challenges brought about by the changes over recent decades in global patterns of living and communication which have political and economic roots.

Beyond such a broad formulation however, more specific explanatory models are needed. Why is it that self-harm has become the response to these challenges? Major social challenges have faced earlier generations and they did not respond in the same way. Without a more detailed explanation of the link, it will always be a struggle to develop effective preventive measures.

Self-harm age and gender

As indicated in Chapter 2, self-harm is rare before puberty. It is commonest in adolescence and young adulthood, when it is 2–3 times commoner among girls and young women than among boys and young men. This is strikingly different to the figures for suicide, which is relatively less common among adolescents and young adults than in middle life; rates for suicide in those aged under 20 are half what they are in the general population and at every age suicide is 2–3 times commoner among males than females (Bachmann, 2018).

Self-harm is the biggest single risk for suicide. Studies show that the suicide rate in the year after a hospital attendance for self-harm is 50 times the general population rate and more than half those who die by suicide have a history of a previous episode of self-harm (Geulayov et al., 2019). And yet the age and sex profiles of the two populations, non-fatal self-harm and suicide, are completely different. Why should this be?

The truth is that this apparent paradox is not fully understood. Some of the reasons that self-harm is so common in young women (high psychological distress, unfavourable gender and social norms, victimization, abuse, and so on) are known but they do not account for all the gender difference (Curtis, 2018; Lutz et al., 2023). And there are some ideas about why men are more at risk of suicide but again they do not explain all the facts. For example, it has been suggested that men are more prone to violent and therefore more dangerous acts of self-harm when they are distressed, but recent figures from the UK show that women who die by suicide are as likely as men to use a method like hanging (Office of National Statistics, 2022). This suggests that there is nothing innately masculine about chosen method of self-harm or suicide, so again we should look for social or cultural explanations.

Negative attitudes

People who self-harm may well be evasive about it. They are worried about the response they will get from those close to them. This sense that self-harm is, despite being so common, something shameful or embarrassing is shared with mental disorders in general and especially other culturally influenced phenomena that have become commoner in recent years—drug and alcohol misuse, gambling, and the emergence of disturbed patterns of eating and weight preoccupation. It is not clear why this should be.

It may be that these problems are commoner in younger people or, as with overweight and self-harm, among females. So perhaps there is a degree of stigma associated with other characteristics that can attract prejudice. Perhaps the common feature is that they are all interpreted as signs of personal weakness, a failure to manage stressful experiences or perhaps to resist temptation.

It is interesting that there are commercial influences on phenomena such as gambling, alcohol use, and dieting so that each of these is seen as socially acceptable in moderation and yet shameful in excess.

The future of sociological research

Despite the obvious importance of social factors in self-harm, sociological research has been much less influential than clinical and psychological research in policy and practice in self-harm.

One reason for this is that it has mainly been rooted in small scale research—in depth qualitative analysis of findings from small numbers of participants. Such research is richly informative in one sense, but it leaves a question about how applicable the findings are at scale. Do they apply to whole populations or substantial sub-populations, or do they not generalize beyond the sample studied?

A second reason is more to do with presentation. Sociological research reports can be quite technical and written for other academics in the field, and it is not easy to see how the findings translate into practical action at the population or public health level where they would be expected to apply.

Self-harm as an individual, psychological phenomenon

Recent efforts have focused on one of two areas:

Given that most of the personal and social problems associated with self-harm are long-standing, a recurrent question (clinical and research) asks—why a particular episode at a particular time? Research to understand the immediate precipitants might lead to new ways of thinking about how to intervene at the right time. Such research can involve new technologies such as experiential momentary sampling techniques/ecological momentary approaches (Gee et al., 2020).

CHAPTER 8

Self-harm is a known risk for suicide. Although we know in general terms what some of the risk factors are for eventual suicide, their predictive value is low. Current research predicting suicide following self-harm has used computer-based models including artificial intelligence (AI) but remains hampered by the fact that although we know many relevant variables any predictive test is likely to struggle when the incidence of the outcome variable (suicide in this case) is low, leading to very high false positive rates.

Intervention research

Clinical provision

There are challenges in providing adequate care after self-harm.

One issue is reluctance on the part of those offered follow-up. This is especially likely among younger people, who may be less willing to confide in an adult whom they see as an authority figure who will judge rather than support them. In many societies men are more reluctant to accept psychological help because they are particularly sensitive to the idea that to do so is a sign of weakness.

Undoubtedly the major barrier, however, is unavailability of suitably trained professionals who can offer relevant support and therapy. The problem is the mismatch between the large numbers of people who self-harm and the much smaller number of professionals able to provide brief therapies. One solution is to increase the availability of peer-support or online resources (see Chapter 7), but for most this theoretical possibility is a long way from reality.

Even when therapeutic interventions are available they cannot be regarded as uniformly successful. We might ask whether there are new therapeutic approaches we ought to develop but it may be better to target existing therapies more effectively rather than develop new ones. For example, social or interpersonal interventions may be more suitable for some people, with more individually focused interventions like cognitive behavioural therapy (CBT) being more applicable for others.

Community level interventions

Even in developed countries, where access to mental health services is much easier than it is in low- and middle-income countries, most people do not access care from a mental health professional after an episode of self-harm. This raises the question of who else might offer support.

For young people there is an obvious answer for those who are still in education or in contact with community support services. Staff in those settings, teachers and social workers, for example, have skills in working with young people and are likely to know at least something about the individual's personal circumstances. The challenge is in knowing what training and support programme is needed, what can be supported given other demands on staff time, and how links to other health and social services can be developed while allowing young people to maintain confidentiality.

CHAPTER 8

The problems that lie behind self-harm are not solely psychological and inter-personal. There are often practical problems related, for example, to debt, em-ployment, housing, or education. Ready access to practical support for these problems can be difficult to arrange. One reason is that their impact results from the interaction between these problems and existing mental health difficulties; the result is that the practical problems when viewed in isolation can seem not that severe and they do not therefore receive the priority they should in societies where many people can be struggling with similar difficulties. This raises a ques-tion about how to prioritize scarce resources.

A particular difficulty is raised by the need to offer accessible services to indi-viduals who are outside conventional social structures, including the homeless or street-connected, young people who have dropped out of education, and those in the criminal justice system. Simple lack of resources is one issue, but lack of resource is compounded by the logistical difficulty of service delivery in settings where there can be high levels of external threat and low levels of trust in official bodies.

Public health

What about preventive programmes? A previous chapter has discussed examples based upon online resources and (for example) in-school programmes (see Chapter 4). As with all preventive efforts there is a question about whether it is more efficient to aim for whole-population coverage or to adopt a strategy of targeting high-risk groups.

Finally, there is a question about the how to develop and support online re-sources to best advantage. Initiatives such as #chatsafe from Australia are encour-aging and to ensure adequate long-term funding and support, this and other schemes need strong evidence of effectiveness.

Notwithstanding the lack of current provision, there are encouraging signs for the future of service development and research as it becomes increasingly clear that self-harm is a near-universal manifestation of distress, understanding and re-sponding to which can be of benefit to a whole society.

In summary

- It is still not clear how to overcome the strong sense of shame and stigma associated with self-harm and its religious, cultural, and social connotations.
- There is a need for more sociological research (to catch up with clinical and psychological research) in influencing policy and practice in self-harm.
- Research is needed to determine whether it is better to target existing interventions more effectively rather than develop new therapeutic approaches.
- Further work is needed to determine how to target resources effectively to tackle the practical problems that lie behind self-harm.

REFERENCES

Aggarwal, S., Patton, G., Reavley, N., Sreenivasan, S. A., & Berk, M. (2017). Youth self-harm in low-and middle-income countries: systematic review of the risk and protective factors. *International Journal of Social Psychiatry*, *63*(4), 359–375. https://doi.org/10.1177/0020764017700175

Bachmann, S. (2018). Epidemiology of suicide and the psychiatric perspective. *International Journal of Environmental Research and Public Health*, *15*(7), 1425. https://doi.org/10.3390/ijerph15071425

Curtis, C. (2018). Female deliberate self-harm: the women's perspectives. *Women's Studies*, *47*(8), 845–867. https://doi.org/10.1080/00497878.2018.1524762

Gee, B. L., Han, J., Benassi, H., & Batterham, P. J. (2020). Suicidal thoughts, suicidal behaviours and self-harm in daily life: a systematic review of ecological momentary assessment studies. *Digital Health*, *6*, 1–38. https://doi.org/10.1177/2055207620963958

Geulayov, G., Casey, D., Bale, L., Brand, F., Clements, C., Farooq, B., Kapur, N., Ness, J., Waters, K., & Tsiachristas, A. (2019). Suicide following presentation to hospital for non-fatal self-harm in the Multicentre Study of Self-harm: a long-term follow-up study. *The Lancet Psychiatry*, *6*(12), 1021–1030. https://doi.org/10.1016/S2215-0366(19)30402-X

Lutz, N. M., Neufeld, S. A., Hook, R. W., Jones, P. B., Bullmore, E. T., Goodyer, I. M., Ford, T. J., Chamberlain, S. R., & Wilkinson, P. O. (2023). Why is non-suicidal self-injury more common in women? Mediation and moderation analyses of psychological distress, emotion dysregulation, and impulsivity. *Archives of Suicide Research*, *27*(3), 905–921. https://doi.org/10.1080/13811118.2022.2084004

Office of National Statistics (2022). *Suicides in England and Wales: 2021 registrations. Registered deaths in England and Wales from suicide analysed by sex, age, area of usual residence of the deceased, and suicide method*. https://www.ons.gov.uk/peoplepopulationandcommunity/birthsdeathsandmarriages/deaths/bulletins/suicidesintheunitedkingdom/2021registrations#suicide-methods

Quarshie, E. N., Waterman, M. G., & House, A. O. (2020). Self-harm with suicidal and non-suicidal intent in young people in sub-Saharan Africa: a systematic review. *BMC Psychiatry*, *20*(1), 1–26. https://doi.org/10.1186/s12888-020-02587-z

Rodway, C., Tham, S.-G., Ibrahim, S., Turnbull, P., Windfuhr, K., Shaw, J., Kapur, N., & Appleby, L. (2016). Suicide in children and young people in England: a consecutive case series. *The Lancet Psychiatry*, *3*(8), 751–759. https://doi.org/10.1016/S2215-0366(16)30094-3

CHAPTER 8

Useful resources and supportive organizations

Books for those affected personally, friends, and family

Books

House, A. (2019). *Understanding and responding to self-harm: the one-stop guide. Practical advice for anybody affected by self-harm.* London: Profile Books Ltd.

House, A., & Brennan, C. (Eds.). (2023). *Social media and mental health.* Cambridge University Press.Selekman, M., & Beyebach, M. (2013). *Changing self-destructive habits: pathways to solutions with couples and families.* New York, NY: Routledge.

Smith, G., Cox, D., & Saradjian, J. (2002). *Women and self harm: understanding, coping and healing from self-mutilation.* Florence, KY: Routledge.

Whitlock, J., & Lloyd-Richardson, E. E. (2019). *Healing self-injury: a compassionate guide for parents and other loved ones.* Oxford University Press.

Supportive organizations

As a global public health challenge, self-harm warrants worldwide and international attention and preventive efforts. Particularly in many high-income countries, national-level organizations and associations exist—bringing together researchers, clinicians and other professionals, advocates, and persons with lived and living experiences to develop self-harm intervention and prevention programmes, such as crisis helpline services, and supportive resources including online resources. These organizations and associations also provide opportunities for networking and volunteering. Notably, however, in low- and middle-income countries the establishment of organizations and associations with a focus on self-harm and suicide intervention and prevention is now emerging. The list provided here is not exhaustive; they are rather indicative.

International supportive organizations

- Befrienders Worldwide: https://befrienders.org/
- International Association for Suicide Prevention (IASP): https://www.iasp.info/
- International Federation of Telephone Emergency Services (IFOTES): https://www.ifotes.org/en

- LifeLine International (LLI): https://lifeline-international.com/
- The International Society for the Study of Self-Injury (ISSS): https://www.itriples.org/
- World Health Organization (WHO): https://www.who.int/

Supportive organizations in high-income countries

- Adolescent Self-Injury Foundation: https://www.adolescentselfinjuryfoundation.com/
- Harmless: https://harmless.org.uk/
- Injury Matters: https://www.injurymatters.org.au/
- Mind: https://www.mind.org.uk/
- National Institute for Health and Care Excellence (NICE): https://www.nice.org.uk/
- Orygen: https://www.orygen.org.au/
- Samaritans: https://www.samaritans.org/
- Self Injury Support Network: https://www.selfinjurysupport.org.uk/
- SelfHarmUK: https://www.selfharm.co.uk/
- Self-injury Outreach and Support (SiOS): https://sioutreach.org/
- Young Minds: https://www.youngminds.org.uk/

Supportive and volunteer organizations in low- and middle-income countries

- **Bangladesh**. Sanity by Tanmoy: https://www.sanitybytanmoy.com/
- **Ghana**. Association for Suicide Prevention Ghana (GASP): https://ghanasp.org/
- **India**. SNEHA: https://snehaindia.org/new/
- **Kenya**. Emergency Medicine Kenya Foundation (https://www.emergencymedicinekenya.org/); CBT Kenya (https://www.cbtkenya.org/our-services/)
- **Namibia**. LifeLine/ChildLine Namibia: https://www.lifelinechildline.org.na/
- **Nigeria**. Nigeria Suicide Prevention: https://nigeriasuicideprevention.com/
- **Pakistan**. Umang Pakistan: https://www.umang.com.pk/
- **South Africa**. The South African Depression and Anxiety Group (SADAG): https://www.sadag.org/
- **Sri Lanka**. Sri Lanka Sumithrayo: https://srilankasumithrayo.lk/
- **Thailand**. The Suicide Prevention in Thailand Project: https://www.suicidethai.com/

- **Uganda**. Uganda Foundation for Suicide Prevention: https://www.ufsp.org/
- **Zambia**. LifeLine ChildLine Zambia: https://clzambia.org/

Online resources

Various resources—including advice, recommendations, and practical informational support to professionals, persons who self-harm or patients and their caretakers, friends, or families—are available online. A recent observational study by Daniel Romeu and colleagues (see: https://www.mdpi.com/1660-4601/17/10/3532) provides a useful annotated list of online resources and a helpful starting point for healthcare professionals wishing to provide some guidance for their patients about using resources available on the internet for self-harm prevention. We agree with the caution by Daniel Romeu and colleagues that as websites change over time and the internet is in constant flux, readers (particularly clinicians) need to review and evaluate online content before making any recommendations to clients or their significant other or families and friends.

Popular online resources for people who self-harm and those involved in their informal and formal care include those provided by:

Orygen: https://www.orygen.org.au/Training/Resources/Self-harm-and-suicide-prevention
SiOS: https://sioutreach.org/
NICE: https://www.nice.org.uk/guidance/ng225
ISSS: https://www.itriples.org/supports
Samaritans: https://www.samaritans.org/how-we-can-help/if-youre-having-difficult-time/if-you-want-self-harm/
Royal College of Psychiatrists: https://www.rcpsych.ac.uk/mental-health/parents-and-young-people/information-for-parents-and-carers/self-harm-for-parents

Index

For the benefit of digital users, indexed terms that span two pages (e.g., 52–53) may, on occasion, appear on only one of those pages.

Tables are indicated by an italic *t* following the page/paragraph number.